Fast Facts

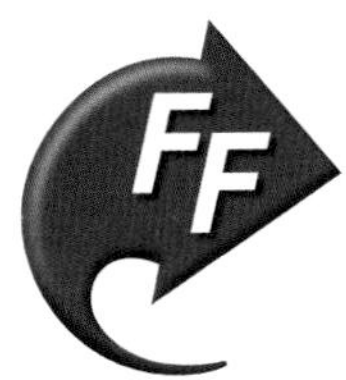

Fast Facts: Prostate Cancer

Eighth edition

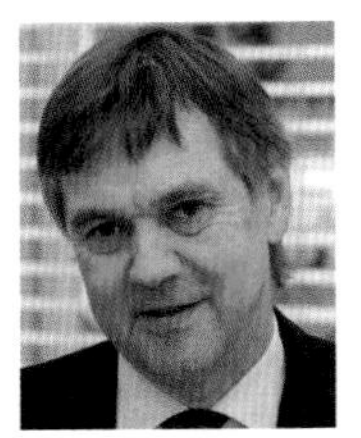

Roger S Kirby MA MD FRCS(Urol) FEBU
Professor of Urology
The Prostate Centre
London, UK

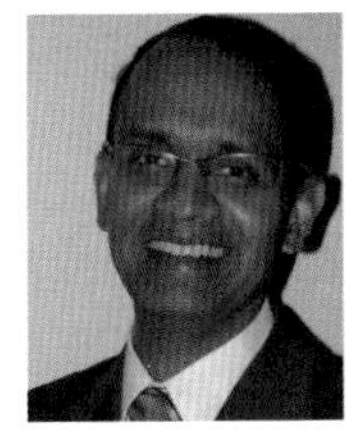

Manish I Patel MBBS MMED PhD FRACS
Associate Professor, University of Sydney
Urological Cancer Surgeon
Westmead Hospital
Sydney, Australia

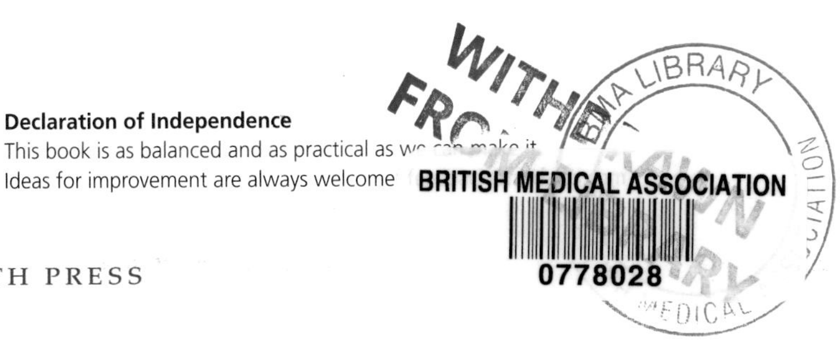

Declaration of Independence
This book is as balanced and as practical as we can make it.
Ideas for improvement are always welcome

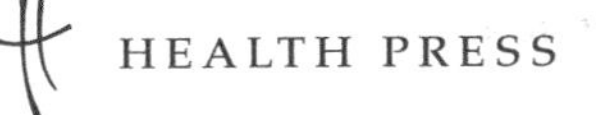

HEALTH PRESS

Fast Facts: Prostate Cancer
First published 1996; second edition 1998; third edition 2001; fourth edition 2004; fifth edition 2008; sixth edition 2009; reprinted 2009, 2010 (thrice); seventh edition 2012

Eighth edition January 2014

Health Press Limited, Elizabeth House, Queen Street, Abingdon, Oxford OX14 3LN, UK
Tel: +44 (0)1235 523233
Fax: +44 (0)1235 523238

Book orders can be placed by telephone or via the website.
For regional distributors or to order via the website, please go to: fastfacts.com
For telephone orders, please call +44 (0)1752 202301 (UK, Europe and Asia–Pacific), 1 800 247 6553 (USA, toll free) or +1 419 281 1802 (Americas).

A CIP record for this title is available from the British Library.

ISBN 978-1-908541-52-9

Kirby RS (Roger)
Fast Facts: Prostate Cancer/
Roger S Kirby, Manish I Patel

Medical illustrations by Dee McLean, London, UK, and Annamaria Dutto, Withernsea, UK.
Typesetting and page layout by Zed, Oxford, UK.
Printed by Latimer Trend & Company Limited, Plymouth, UK.

Text printed with vegetable inks on biodegradable and recyclable paper manufactured using elemental chlorine free (ECF) wood pulp from well-managed forests.

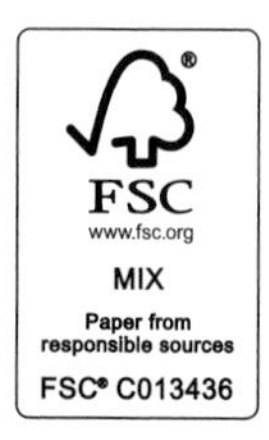

Glossary and abbreviations

5α-reductase: the enzyme that converts testosterone to DHT

Antiandrogens: drugs that compete with testosterone or its metabolite DHT for binding to androgen receptors in the prostate

BPH: benign prostatic hyperplasia

Brachytherapy: interstitial radiotherapy

Chemoprevention: the use of drugs to reduce the risk of cancer

CRPC: castrate-resistant prostate cancer

Cryoablation: the use of freezing temperatures to destroy tissue

CT: computerized tomography

DES: diethylstilbestrol

DHT: dihydrotestosterone

DRE: digital rectal examination

HDR brachytherapy: high-dose-rate brachytherapy

HIFU: high-intensity focused ultrasound

LHRH: luteinizing hormone-releasing hormone

LHRH agonists: LHRH analogs are used to achieve androgen deprivation by inducing chemical castration. They initially stimulate the anterior pituitary resulting in a transient increase in testosterone

LHRH antagonists: pure antagonists that shut off LHRH release, obviating the flare phenomenon seen with LHRH agonists

MRI: magnetic resonance imaging

PET: positron emission tomography

PSA: prostate-specific antigen

TGF: transforming growth factor

TNM: tumor–nodes–metastasis (a staging system for cancer)

TRUS: transrectal ultrasonography

TURP: transurethral resection of the prostate

Introduction

It has aptly been said that we are all drowning in a sea of information, but thirsting for knowledge. In this concise handbook, we summarize our current knowledge of the most common cancer in men. Prostate cancer continues to take a significant toll on human health and happiness. It's certainly not a good condition to have, but recent advances have significantly improved not only the survival prospects, but also the quality of life, of many men diagnosed with this disease. This eighth edition of *Fast Facts: Prostate Cancer* aims to set out lucidly, and in an evidence-based fashion, all these new developments and to put them in context.

Prostate cancer is common. There is now a one in eight chance of a man developing the disease. More than 45 000 men will be diagnosed in the UK this year, and more than ten times that number in the USA. Worldwide, many hundreds of thousands of men are destined to die each year from this cancer. The good news is that more and more men will survive for longer periods after diagnosis, largely because of recent advances in management. This, of course, raises important 'survivorship' issues, and we cover these in a new chapter.

Other advances are also covered in this new edition. For example, the molecular basis of prostate cancer is now coming more clearly into focus. Rather like the estrogen receptor in breast cancer, the androgen receptor is central to the pathogenesis of prostate cancer. Receptor mutations that promote tumor cell division appear to underlie the development of castrate-resistant prostate cancer.

Controversy still swirls around the issue of prostate-specific antigen (PSA) screening. While PSA is insufficiently robust for population-based screening, sequential PSA measurements over time, plus 3-Tesla multiparametric MRI, can unquestionably save lives in some circumstances. Better diagnostic markers are also now on the horizon, as well as new information on chemoprevention.

Genetic markers are now emerging that look promising as clinical tools to identify men who need treatment and distinguish them from those who can be simply monitored in an active surveillance program.

In time, these markers may compliment or even replace the current PSA test and Gleason scoring system as prognostic tools.

The treatment of clinically localized disease remains contentious. Evidence is mounting that around two-thirds of men with so-called 'low-risk' disease will never need treatment and can be safely monitored with PSA, MRI and occasional re-biopsy.

For those with higher-risk, but still localized, disease, debate about the merits of surgery versus radiotherapy is ongoing. We have updated the treatment sections to include information about robot-assisted surgery and the newer methods of delivering radiotherapy, such as low-dose seed brachytherapy and CyberKnife.

New and more effective methods of dealing with castrate-resistant cancer have emerged: taxane-based chemotherapy with either docetaxel or cabazitaxel has been shown to prolong survival and improve quality of life. Abiraterone has been shown to be effective, used either before or after chemotherapy. And enzalutamide, another compound supported by encouraging results, has been approved for similar use, but currently only after chemotherapy. We look at how these therapies fit into treatment options for patients.

We hope that, through this book, we can make a useful contribution toward enhancing the knowledge of all those who provide support and care for men with prostate cancer, including GPs, nurses and allied healthcare professionals. Our ultimate aim is to improve the care and survivorship of those very many men who have recently been, or are destined to be, diagnosed with and treated for this most prevalent disease.

1 Epidemiology and pathophysiology

In most developed and, increasingly, in developing countries, prostate cancer is the most common malignancy to affect men of middle age and beyond, and is second only to lung cancer as a cause of cancer deaths in men. It has been estimated that, in western countries, the lifetime risk of developing microscopic prostate cancer is 30%. At autopsy, the prevalence of microscopic prostate cancer is approximately 80% in men aged 80 years. However, as many of these cancers grow slowly, the risk of developing clinically detectable cancer is about 8%; the lifetime risk of actually dying from prostate cancer is approximately 3%.

Worldwide, there has been a steady increase in the incidence of clinically significant disease but, in the USA at least, the data indicate that incidence is now plateauing (Figure 1.1). However, because

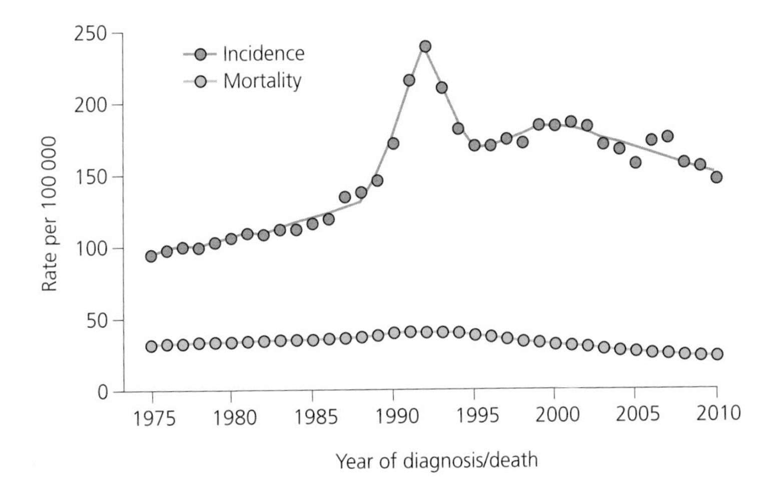

Figure 1.1 The incidence and mortality for prostate cancer in the USA from 1975 to 2010. A temporary rise in incidence was noted with the introduction of prostate-specific antigen (PSA) screening. Data are from the US National Cancer Institute (NCI) Surveillance Epidemiology and End Results (SEER; http://seer.cancer.gov/data).

prostate cancer is primarily a disease affecting men over the age of 50 years, the worldwide trend towards an aging population means that the number of men diagnosed with prostate cancer is predicted to increase substantially over the next two decades. Mortality from prostate cancer in Europe rose to a peak in 1993, reached a plateau, and has now started to decrease. Mortality in the USA has recently shown similar trends and has also started to decline (see Figure 1.1). The rate of decline has increased significantly in recent years and is now four times faster than the rate in the UK. Some have attributed this drop to the efforts made in North America to detect prostate cancer early, though several other factors such as changes in lifestyle and better treatment outcomes may also have contributed.

Risk factors

Despite the high incidence of prostate cancer, relatively little is known about the underlying causes of the disease. However, a number of risk factors have been established (Table 1.1).

Age is the greatest factor influencing the development of prostate cancer. Clinical disease is rare in men under the age of 50 years, and the incidence increases markedly in men over 60 years of age (Figure 1.2).

Race. There are marked geographic and ethnic variations in the incidence of clinical prostate cancer (see, for example, Figure 1.2). The risk is highest in North America and northern European

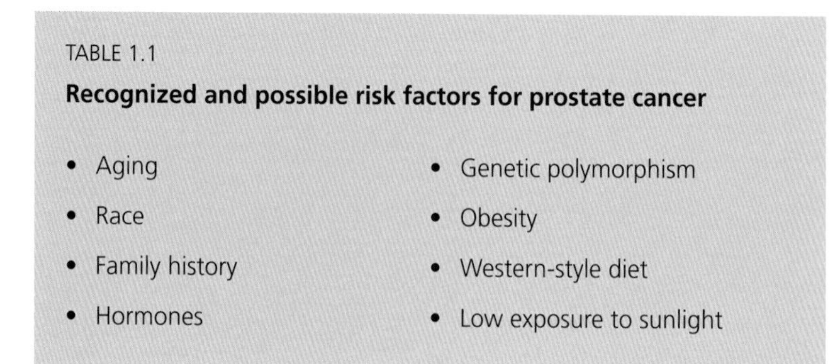
TABLE 1.1

Recognized and possible risk factors for prostate cancer

- Aging
- Race
- Family history
- Hormones
- Genetic polymorphism
- Obesity
- Western-style diet
- Low exposure to sunlight

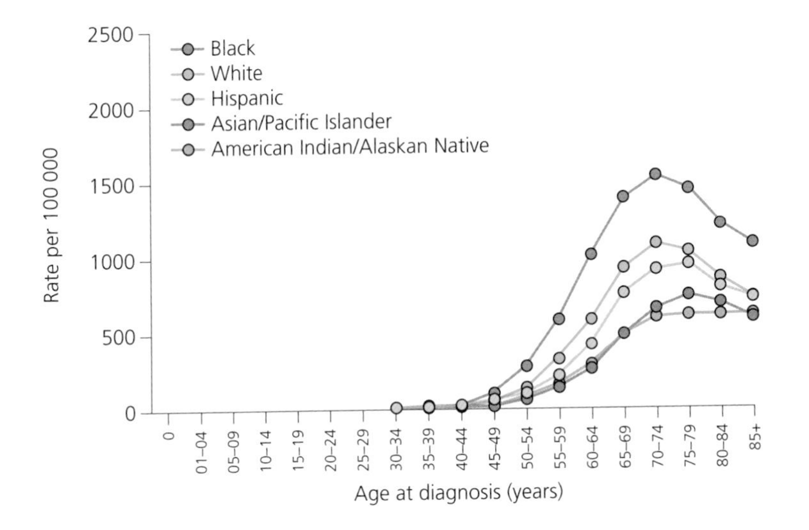

Figure 1.2 Age-specific incidence of prostate cancer by race in the USA from 1992 to 2010 (pooled data). Data are from the US National Cancer Institute Surveillance Epidemiology and End Results (SEER; http://seer.cancer.gov/data).

countries, and lowest in the Far East. In the USA, the risk is higher in blacks than in whites, and black men also appear to develop more aggressive disease earlier. Chinese and Japanese races show the lowest incidence of prostate cancer, though the prevalence is now increasing in both. The incidence of latent, clinically insignificant disease, however, is similar in all populations studied. In migration studies, the incidence of prostate cancer in men emigrating from a low- to a high-risk area increases to that of the local population within two generations. This suggests that environmental influences such as diet and nutrition may have a profound effect on the development of prostate cancer and on the progression of histological cancer to a clinically detectable cancer.

Family history/genetic risk. Overall, epidemiologic studies show that heritable factors account for a small proportion of prostate cancer risk, but a higher proportion of early-onset disease. However, the existence of prostate cancer susceptibility genes is suggested by a host of studies, and family history is a strong risk factor for prostate cancer. The risk of a man developing prostate cancer if he has a first-degree relative affected is increased approximately 2.5-fold. The relative risks for developing prostate cancer based on family history are given in Table 1.2.

Linkage analyses, which screen for genetic traits in high-risk groups in whom prostate cancer has been detected, have identified many prostate cancer susceptibility loci (physical locations of genes/DNA on a chromosome). However, the high 'background' incidence of sporadic prostate cancers can make statistical analyses of these results difficult. It appears that many of the loci are associated with cancer in a small group of families, and currently there is no single genetic marker that indicates increased susceptibility to prostate cancer. Researchers are looking at combining single nucleotide polymorphisms in multiplex

TABLE 1.2

Risk of developing prostate cancer in relation to family history of the disease

Family history	Relative risk (95% CI)
≥ 2 first-degree relatives diagnosed at any age	4.39 (2.61, 7.39)
Brother(s) diagnosed at any age	3.14 (2.37, 4.15)
First-degree relative diagnosed < 65 years	2.87 (2.21, 3.74)
Second-degree relatives diagnosed at any age	2.52 (0.99, 6.46)
First-degree relative diagnosed at any age	2.48 (2.25, 2.74)
Father diagnosed at any age	2.35 (2.02, 2.72)
First-degree relative diagnosed ≥ 65 years	1.92 (1.49, 2.47)

CI, confidence interval.
Adapted from Kiciński M et al., 2011.

assays, but more research is needed before tests become routinely available. The US National Cancer Institute's webpages on the genetics of prostate cancer are regularly updated and provide a thorough review of the current status of this fast-changing field (www.cancer.gov/cancertopics/pdq/genetics/prostate).

Mutations in the *BRCA* breast cancer susceptibility genes are rare in men with prostate cancer, but appear to be associated with features of more aggressive disease, such as higher Gleason score, and higher PSA level and tumor stage and/or grade at diagnosis. Furthermore, carriers of *BRCA* mutations may have lower overall survival and prostate cancer-specific survival compared with non-carriers. Knowledge of a man's *BRCA* status is, therefore, of prognostic value.

Hormones. Testosterone and its more potent metabolite dihydrotestosterone (DHT) are essential for normal prostate growth and also play a role in the development of prostate cancer (Figure 1.3). Prostate cancer almost never develops in the rare men castrated before puberty, or in men deficient in 5α-reductase (the enzyme, existing in type I and II isoforms, that converts testosterone to DHT). Trials of

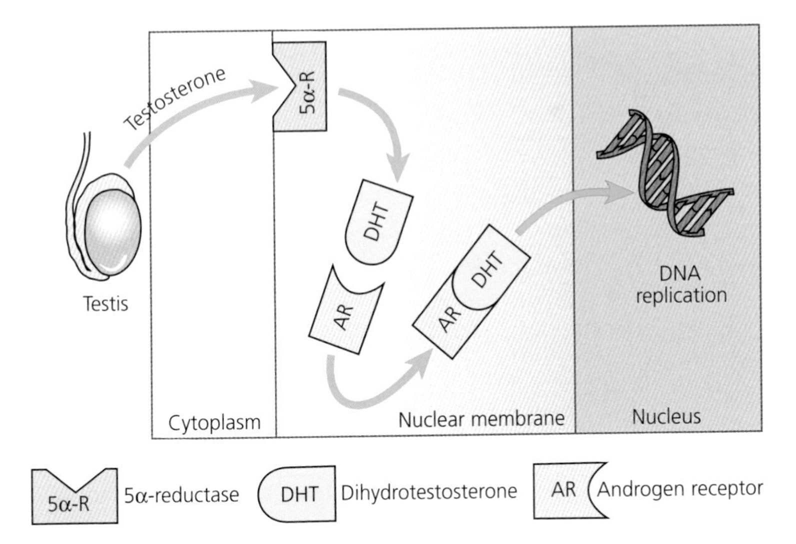

Figure 1.3 Testosterone, which is converted to DHT by 5α-reductase, supports prostate cell function and stimulates cell division.

type II 5α-reductase inhibition with finasteride and dutasteride have shown that the development of prostate cancer can be reduced by around 25%, suggesting a key role for DHT. However, the incidence of prostate cancer increases with age, while serum testosterone levels decrease. In addition, men diagnosed with advanced prostate cancer often have a lower average testosterone level than men of a similar age who do not have prostate cancer.

Obesity. The suggested link between body mass index and incidence of prostate cancer has been controversial. Early studies showed an increased risk of prostate cancer in obese men, while more recent studies have suggested that obese men actually have lower levels of detected prostate cancer. This may be because levels of PSA and androgens are lower in obese men, so fewer obese men may be being biopsied and diagnosed with prostate cancer in the PSA era. There is, however, a clear increase in prostate cancer mortality in men who are obese. The mechanism by which obesity increases the likelihood of death from prostate cancer is not known; it may be through the activation of pro-carcinogenic pathways such as the insulin-like growth factor (IGF) axis.

Western diets are high in animal fat, protein, meat and processed carbohydrates, and low in plant foods. A link between dietary fat, saturated fat and meat intake and the development of prostate cancer has been supported by a number of studies. There is also some evidence that α-linoleic acid, an omega-3 polyunsaturated fatty acid, increases prostate cancer risk and the risk of developing advanced prostate cancer. This may be the result of oxidative stress and subsequent DNA damage or the development of obesity. Omega-3 fatty acids from marine sources may result in a decreased risk of developing prostate cancer.

Sun exposure and vitamin D. The risk of dying from prostate cancer is geographically related to ultraviolet (UV) light exposure. Vitamin D levels in men with prostate cancer are lower than in men without, and vitamin D levels are determined by dietary intake and conversion in the skin by UV light. The mechanism by which vitamin D levels protect against prostate cancer is not known. Calcitriol (vitamin D) has been used to treat advanced prostate cancer, but evidence of efficacy is lacking.

Histological features

Most prostate cancers are adenocarcinomas that appear to arise in the peripheral zone of the gland (> 70%) (Figure 1.4). Approximately

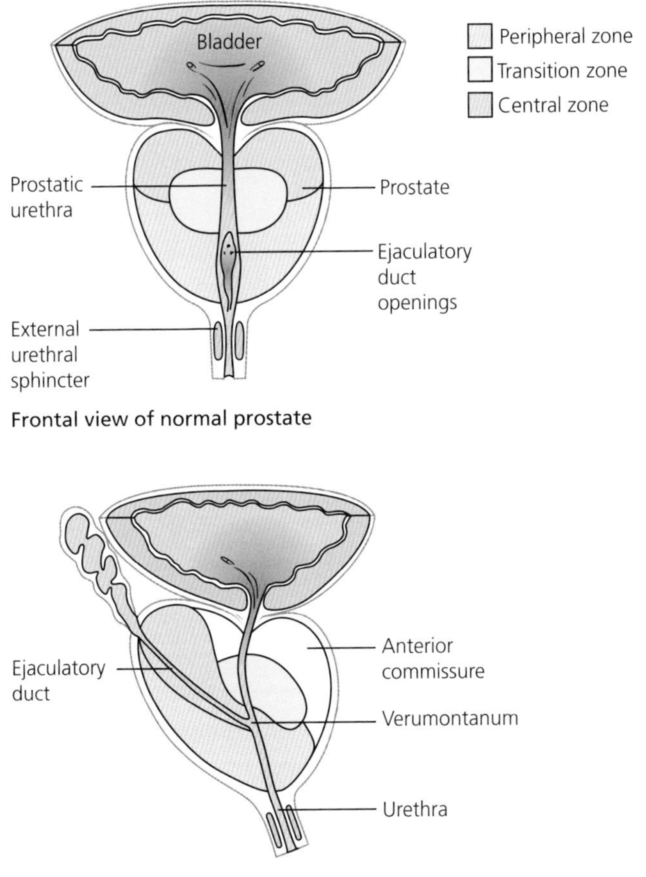

Figure 1.4 Approximately 70% of prostate cancers arise in the peripheral zone.

5–15% arise in the central zone and the remainder from the transition zone, which is the zone where benign prostatic hyperplasia (BPH) also develops.

Microscopic foci of 'latent' prostate cancer are a common autopsy finding and may appear very early in life; approximately 30% of men over 50 years of age have evidence of latent disease. Because of the very slow growth rate of these microscopic tumors, many never progress to clinical disease. Beyond a certain size, however, these lesions progressively de-differentiate, probably owing to clonal selection, and become increasingly invasive. A tumor that has a volume greater than 0.5 cm^3 or is anything other than well differentiated is generally regarded as clinically significant.

The Gleason system is the most widely used system for grading prostate cancer (Figure 1.5). It recognizes five levels of increasing aggressiveness.

- Grade 1 tumors consist of small, uniform glands with minimal nuclear changes.
- Grade 2 tumors have medium-sized acini, still separated by stromal tissue, but more closely arranged.
- Grade 3 tumors, the most common finding, show marked variation in glandular size and organization, and general infiltration of stromal and neighboring tissues.
- Grade 4 tumors show marked cytological atypia with extensive infiltration.
- Grade 5 tumors are characterized by sheets of undifferentiated cancer cells.

Because prostate cancers are often heterogeneous, the numbers of the two most widely represented grades are added together to produce the Gleason score (e.g. 3 + 4). This score (or sum) provides useful prognostic information; Gleason scores above 4 are associated with a progressive risk of more rapid disease progression, increased metastatic potential and decreased survival (Table 1.3). A meta-analysis of patients being managed by active surveillance/watchful waiting (the distinction between the two approaches, as described later, was not clear in the paper), for example, found that the annual

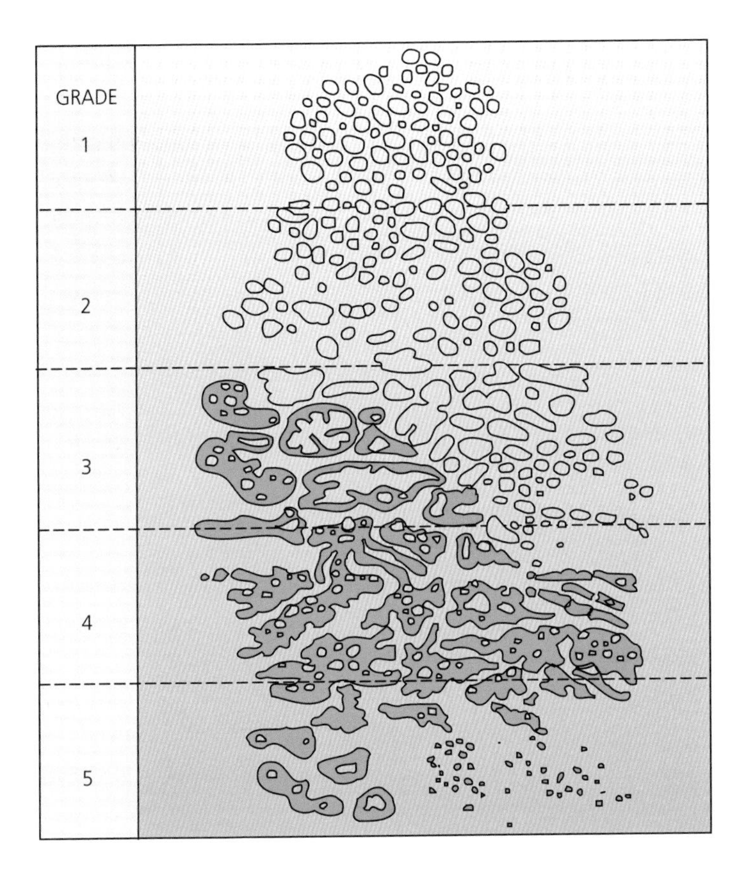

Figure 1.5 The Gleason grading system is based on the extent to which the tumor cells are arranged into recognizably glandular structures. Grade 1 tumors form almost normal glands that are progressively lost through the grades. By grade 5, tumors are characterized by sheets of undifferentiated cancer cells. In individual patients, the prognosis worsens with the progressive loss of glandular differentiation. Because prostate cancers are often heterogeneous in histological pattern, the Gleason score (or sum) is calculated by the summation of the grades of the two predominant areas. Adapted from Gleason DF. The Veterans' Administration Cooperative Urologic Research Group: Histologic grading and clinical staging of prostatic carcinoma. In: Tannenbaum M, ed. *Urologic Pathology: The Prostate*. Philadelphia: Lea and Febiger, 1977:171–98.

TABLE 1.3
The Gleason score*

Gleason score	Histological characteristics	10-year likelihood of local progression (%)
2–6	Well differentiated	25
7	Moderately differentiated	50
8–10	Poorly differentiated	75

*The Gleason score is the sum of the two most prominent grades.

rate of developing metastases was 2.1% in patients with Gleason scores below 4, compared with 5.4% in patients with scores between 5 and 7, and 13.5% in patients with scores above 7. The chance of relapse after radical prostatectomy has also been shown to be directly proportional to the percentage of Gleason grade 4 and 5 cancer in the specimen. Occasionally, more than two grades are observed in prostatectomy specimens, the least common being known as the tertiary grade. When the tertiary grade has a high score (4 or 5), the patient has a higher risk of progression, even if the primary and secondary grades are lower.

One study of 767 men with localized prostate cancer reported a highly significant correlation between the Gleason score and the risk of dying from prostate cancer. Patients with a score of 2–4 had a 4–7% chance of dying within 15 years of diagnosis. In contrast, patients with a score of 8–10 had a 60–87% chance of death from prostate cancer.

Patterns of disease spread

Prostate cancer can be classified according to the spread of the disease by the tumor–nodes–metastasis (TNM) system (Table 1.4). The tumor stage (T1–T4) describes the pathological development of the tumor.

- T1 represents 'incidental' status, in which the tumor is discovered after transurethral resection of the prostate (TURP) or, more commonly, by PSA testing, and is not detectable by palpation or ultrasonography.

TABLE 1.4

The TNM classification of prostate cancer (2010)

Primary tumor

Category	Subcategory	Description
Tx		Primary tumor cannot be assessed
T0		No evidence of primary tumor
T1		Clinically inapparent tumor not palpable or visible by imaging
	T1a	Incidental; histological finding in ≤ 5% of tissue resected
	T1b	Incidental; histological finding in > 5% of tissue resected
	T1c	Identified by needle biopsy (e.g. because of elevated PSA)
T2		Tumor confined within the prostate*
	T2a	Involves ≤ 50% of one lobe
	T2b	Involves > 50% of one lobe but not both lobes
	T2c	Involves both lobes
T3		Tumor extends through the prostatic capsule[†]
	T3a	Extracapsular extension (unilateral or bilateral)
	T3b	Invades seminal vesicle(s)
T4		Tumor is fixed or invades adjacent structures other than seminal vesicles: bladder neck, external sphincter, rectum, levator muscles and/or pelvic wall

Regional lymph nodes

Nx	Cannot be assessed
N0	No metastasis
N1	Metastasis

Distant metastasis[‡]

Category	Subcategory	Description
Mx		Cannot be assessed
M0		No metastasis
M1		Metastasis
	M1a	Non-regional lymph node(s)
	M1b	Bone(s)
	M1c	Other site(s)

*Tumor found in one or both lobes by needle biopsy, but not palpable or visible by imaging, is classified as T1c.
[†]Invasion into the prostatic apex or into (but not beyond) the prostatic capsule is not classified as T3, but as T2.
[‡]When ≥1 site of metastasis, the most advanced category should be used.
TNM, tumor–nodes–metastasis.

- T2 represents a cancer which is palpable but still confined to the prostate gland.
- T3 represents a cancer which has extended through the prostate capsule into the surrounding fat or seminal vesicles.
- T4 represents advanced disease, in which the tumor invades neighboring organs (Figure 1.6).

The nodal stages (N0–N1) and metastatic stages (M0–M1c) reflect the clinical progression of the disease. Metastases are most common in the lymph nodes (N1) and bones (M1); the lungs and other soft tissues are less commonly involved.

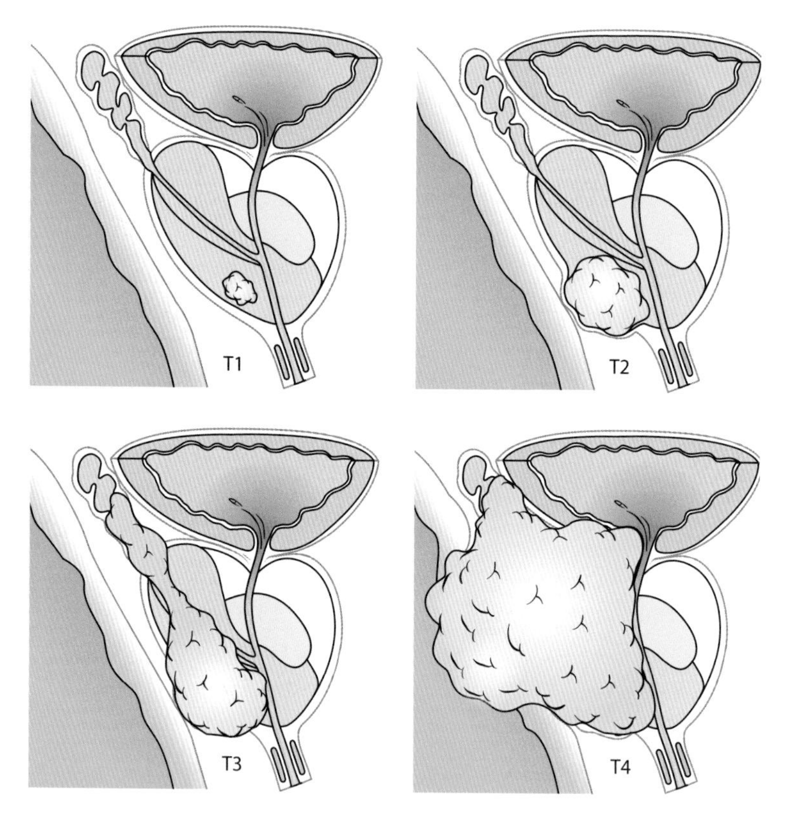

Figure 1.6 The tumor–nodes–metastasis (TNM) system recognizes four stages of local tumor growth: T1 (incidental); T2 (confined within the prostate); T3 (extending through the prostatic capsule); and T4 (invading neighboring organs).

Currently, it is not possible to distinguish unambiguously between those tumors that will remain latent throughout the patient's life and those that will definitely progress to clinical disease. Studies of incidental carcinomas diagnosed after TURP suggest that the median time to progression for T1b (high-volume, moderately or poorly differentiated) tumors is 4.75 years, compared with 13.5 years for T1a (low-volume, well-differentiated) tumors (Figure 1.7). Thus, elderly men with T1a tumors are more appropriately managed by active surveillance alone, while younger men with T1b disease may be considered, after informed consent, for more aggressive, potentially curative therapy.

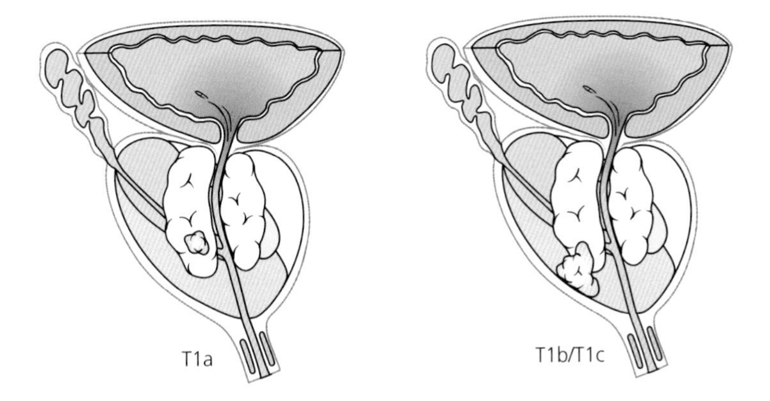

Figure 1.7 Incidental carcinoma of the prostate is unsuspected cancer diagnosed at transurethral resection of the prostate. T1a cancers are small, well-differentiated lesions involving less than 5% of resected tissue. T1b cancers are larger, involve more than 5% of the resected chippings and are less well differentiated. T1c cancers detected by PSA testing are usually greater than 0.5 cm^3 in volume and moderately well differentiated. TURP, transurethral resection of the prostate.

Key points – epidemiology and pathophysiology

- Prostate cancer is soon likely to become the most common cause of cancer death in men.
- Age is the greatest risk factor, but race, family history, western-style diet and obesity also have an effect.
- Most prostate cancers are adenocarcinomas arising in the peripheral zone of the gland.
- Prostate cancers are graded according to the Gleason system, which carries prognostic significance.

Key references

Albertsen PC, Hanley JA, Fine J. 20-year outcomes following conservative management of clinically localized prostate cancer. *JAMA* 2005;293:2095–101.

Andriole GL, Bostwick DG, Brawley OW et al. Effect of dutasteride on the risk of prostate cancer. *N Engl J Med* 2010;362:1192–202.

Calle EE, Rodriguez C, Walker-Thurmond K, Thun MJ. Overweight, obesity, and mortality from cancer in a prospectively studied cohort of U.S. adults. *N Engl J Med* 2003;348:1625–38.

Chen C. Risk of prostate cancer in relation to polymorphisms of metabolic genes. *Epidemiol Rev* 2001;23:30–5.

Giovannucci E, Liu Y, Platz EA et al. Risk factors for prostate cancer incidence and progression in the health professionals follow-up study. *Int J Cancer* 2007;121:1571–8.

Kiciński M, Vangronsveld J, Nawrot TS. An epidemiological reappraisal of the familial aggregation of prostate cancer: a meta-analysis. *PLoS One* 2011;6:e27130.

Langeberg WJ, Isaacs WB, Stanford JL. Genetic etiology of hereditary prostate cancer. *Front Biosci* 2007;12:4101–10.

Leitzmann MF, Stampfer MJ, Michaud DS et al. Dietary intake of n-3 and n-6 fatty acids and the risk of prostate cancer. *Am J Clin Nutr* 2004;80:204–16.

Mitra AV, Bancroft EK, Barbachano Y et al. Targeted prostate cancer screening in men with mutations in *BRCA1* and *BRCA2* detects aggressive prostate cancer: preliminary analysis of the results of the IMPACT study. *BJU Int* 2011;107:28–39.

Moyad MA. Lifestyle/dietary supplement partial androgen suppression and/or estrogen manipulation. A novel PSA reducer and preventive/treatment option for prostate cancer? *Urol Clin North Am* 2002;29:115–24.

Thompson IM, Goodman PJ, Tangen CM et al. The influence of finasteride on the development of prostate cancer. *N Engl J Med* 2003;349:215–24.

Zheng SL, Sun J, Wiklund F et al. Cumulative association of five genetic variants with prostate cancer. *N Engl J Med* 2008;358:910–19.

Effect on development of prostate cancer

Diet and lifestyle are clearly linked to the development of prostate cancer. In Chapter 1, the effect of hormones, obesity and a western-

TABLE 2.1

Effects of dietary manipulation to reduce the incidence of prostate cancer

Compound	Source	Maximum suggested effect
Calcium	• Dietary supplement • Dairy products	• Reported to increase risk by up to 70% in some studies
Fish oils	• Oily fish	• Conflicting data: recent SELECT study suggested 43% increased risk in men with highest blood levels of omega-3 fatty acids
Lycopene	• Tomatoes • Watermelon • Pink grapefruit • Guava	• 15–20% reduction, increasing to 25% if > 2 servings of tomato product/week
Saturated fat	• Saturated fats, including red meat and dairy	• 10–30% increase
Selenium	• Grains • Fish • Meat • Poultry • Dairy products	• Approximately 50% reduction with 200 μg daily in some studies • Excessive intake can be toxic
Soy/ isoflavonoids	• Soy products	• Up to 70% reduction if > 1 serving of soy milk daily
Vitamin D	• Supplements • Sunlight	• Not established
Vitamin E	• Supplements	• Approximately 30% reduction with 50 mg daily
Zinc	• Dietary supplements	• Not established but concerns that supplements may increase risk

style diet were discussed as risk factors for the development of prostate cancer. A large number of studies have evaluated the effects of dietary manipulation/supplementation or drug treatment to reduce the incidence of prostate cancer. Table 2.1 shows the current evidence for dietary manipulation.

Although randomized clinical trials have provided some indication of a protective effect from selenium and vitamin E, a large

Strength of evidence	Comment
Medium	• Conflicting study results but many also show no increased risk
Medium	• SELECT study did not assess participants' diet or use of supplements. Other studies suggest omega-3 fatty acids from marine sources have a protective role. No clear conclusions can be drawn at present.
Medium	• Better effect with cooked or processed tomato products (e.g. tomato sauce)
Poor	• Associations with total fat, saturated fat, meat and linoleic acid have been reported
Medium	• Some evidence of effect, particularly in those with low PSA levels and low plasma selenium levels, but results from large randomized controlled trial were disappointing
Medium	• No strong evidence but lower level evidence consistently supports an effect
Poor	• No substantial evidence to support an effect
Medium	• Some suggestion of an effect, but results from large randomized controlled trial were disappointing
Poor	• Epidemiological and experimental data are conflicting

Strength of evidence: Medium, single-arm study; Poor, anecdotal.

chemoprevention study (the Selenium and Vitamin E Cancer Prevention Trial [SELECT]), designed to determine whether they reduced the likelihood of prostate cancer when used singly or in combination, was ended prematurely because of disappointingly negative results. Cohort studies show that lycopene and isoflavonoids – in, respectively, tomatoes and soy products – are possibly associated with a decrease in the incidence of prostate cancer. Evidence for other dietary supplements is weak.

Chemoprevention with drugs. The 5α-reductase inhibitor finasteride has been shown to reduce the incidence of prostate cancer by 24.8% compared with placebo over a 7-year period, though at the cost of a small incidence of sexual side effects. Counterbalancing this observation is the finding that a small proportion of the cancers in the finasteride group tended to be more aggressive in nature than those in the placebo group. The explanation for this is still debated, but it is possibly explained by an artifact of biopsying the smaller prostates that resulted from the shrinkage effect of finasteride in the active treatment arm of the study. A recent report has confirmed no difference in the rates of overall survival, or survival after a diagnosis of prostate cancer, between the placebo-treated and finasteride-treated patients after 18 years of follow-up.

Another 5α-reductase inhibitor, dutasteride, has been evaluated for its effect on the occurrence of prostate cancer in the so-called REDUCE study (Reduction by Dutasteride of Prostate Cancer Events). Dutasteride resulted in a 23% reduction in prostate cancer risk, mainly by suppressing the well-differentiated cancers, with only a slight, statistically insignificant, increase in Gleason pattern 7 or 8–10 poorly differentiated tumors. It also effectively treated the symptoms arising from benign prostatic enlargement in participants.

Significantly, neither of these compounds has been approved by the regulatory authorities for chemoprevention.

Recently, statins have been reported to have some chemopreventative properties. Evidence for this is still weak but it is an intriguing possibility.

Effect on progression

Unfortunately, very few clinical trials have investigated the effect of diet and lifestyle change on prostate cancer progression. Table 2.2 outlines the current body of evidence. In addition to this, a large number of compounds – many of them herbal – have been tested in the laboratory and show possible promise; these include green tea and other polyphenols, resveratrol from red wine, vitamin D, epilobium and *Serenoa repens* (saw palmetto).

TABLE 2.2

Effect of diet and lifestyle on prostate cancer progression

Factor and effect	Comment
Exercise	
No clear evidence but suspected to be of benefit	Performance index is an independent prognostic indicator in clinical trials
Low-fat diet	
Possible reduction in cancer growth	Low level of clinical benefit based on animal and human biomarker studies
Fish oils/omega-3 fatty acids	
Possible reduction in cancer growth	Based on a cohort study and an animal study
Lycopene	
Reasonable evidence of a reduction in PSA and tumor size	2 servings per week associated with 20% risk reduction from cohort and animal studies
Pomegranate juice	
Possible reduction in PSA rise after prostate cancer recurrence	Based on low-level evidence from phase II trials
Soy/isoflavonoids	
Inconclusive evidence of any benefit	In-vitro results favorable but an animal study was not supportive

It must be remembered that the major killer in men with or without prostate cancer is cardiovascular disease. To reduce mortality in men with prostate cancer, heart-healthy lifestyle choices must be made. These include improving lipid profiles, decreasing obesity and increasing physical fitness. Not only will these measures decrease the risk of death from cardiovascular causes, but a healthy diet and regular vigorous exercise may help defend the individual against various forms of cancer as well.

Key points – diet, lifestyle and chemoprevention

- In a trial, dutasteride reduced the incidence of prostate cancer by about one-quarter over 4 years and also treated benign prostatic hyperplasia symptoms, but slightly increased the incidence of high-grade cancer. Finasteride produced similar results.
- Men should be advised/supported to lower lipid profiles, decrease obesity and increase fitness as part of a strategy to cut the risk of cardiovascular disease and, possibly, prostate cancer.

Key references

Andriole GL, Bostwick DG, Brawley OW et al. Effect of dutasteride on the risk of prostate cancer. *N Engl J Med* 2010;362: 1192–202.

Brasky TM, Darke AK, Song X et al. Plasma phospholipid fatty acids and prostate cancer risk in the SELECT trial. *J Natl Cancer Inst* 2013;105: 1132–41.

Cohen YC, Liu KS, Heyden NL et al. Detection bias due to the effect of finasteride on prostate volume: a modeling approach for analysis of the Prostate Cancer Prevention Trial. *J Natl Cancer Inst* 2007;99: 1366–74.

Duffield-Lillico AJ, Dalkin BL, Reid ME et al. Selenium supplementation, baseline plasma selenium status and incidence of prostate cancer: an analysis of the complete treatment period of the Nutritional Prevention of Cancer Trial. *BJU Int* 2003;91:608–12.

Giovannucci E, Liu Y, Platz EA et al. Risk factors for prostate cancer incidence and progression in the health professionals follow-up study. *Int J Cancer* 2007;121:1571–8.

Gomella L. Chemoprevention using dutasteride: the REDUCE trial. *Curr Opin Urol* 2005;15:29–32.

Lippmani SM, Klein EA, Goodman PJ et al. Effect of selenium and vitamin E on risk of prostate cancer and other cancers: the Selenium and Vitamin E Cancer Prevention Trial (SELECT). *JAMA* 2009;301:39–51.

Lucia MS, Epstein JI, Goodman PJ et al. Finasteride and high-grade prostate cancer in the Prostate Cancer Prevention Trial. *J Natl Cancer Inst* 2007;99:1375–83.

Miller EC, Giovannucci E, Erdman JW Jr et al. Tomato products, lycopene, and prostate cancer risk. *Urol Clin North Am* 2002;29:83–93.

Shepherd BE, Redman MW, Ankerst DP. Does finasteride affect the severity of prostate cancer? A causal sensitivity analysis. *J Am Stat Assoc* 2008;103:1392–404.

Thompson IM, Chi C, Ankerst DP et al. Effect of finasteride on the sensitivity of PSA for detecting prostate cancer. *J Natl Cancer Inst* 2006;98:1128–33.

Thompson IM, Goodman PJ, Tangen CM et al. The influence of finasteride on the development of prostate cancer. *N Engl J Med* 2003;349:215–24.

Thompson IM, Goodman PJ, Tangen CM et al. Long-term survival in the Prostate Cancer Prevention Trial. *N Engl J Med* 2013;369:603–10.

Virtamo J, Pietinen P, Huttunen JK et al. Incidence of cancer and mortality following alpha-tocopherol and beta-carotene supplementation: a postintervention follow-up. *JAMA* 2003;290:476–85.

3 Screening and early detection

The past decade has seen a significant downward shift in the stage at presentation of prostate cancer in most countries. Historically, most men with significant disease presented with a combination of weight loss, bone pain, lethargy and bladder outflow obstruction attributable to locally advanced or metastatic disease. Increasingly, however, early disease is detected incidentally using measurement of prostate-specific antigen (PSA) in younger, asymptomatic patients; occasionally it is an incidental histological finding following a transurethral resection of the prostate (TURP) for benign obstructive symptoms. This earlier presentation has posed dilemmas concerning management, and the increasing life expectancy of patients (Figure 3.1) underscores the urgent need for effective evidence-based diagnosis and treatment regimens.

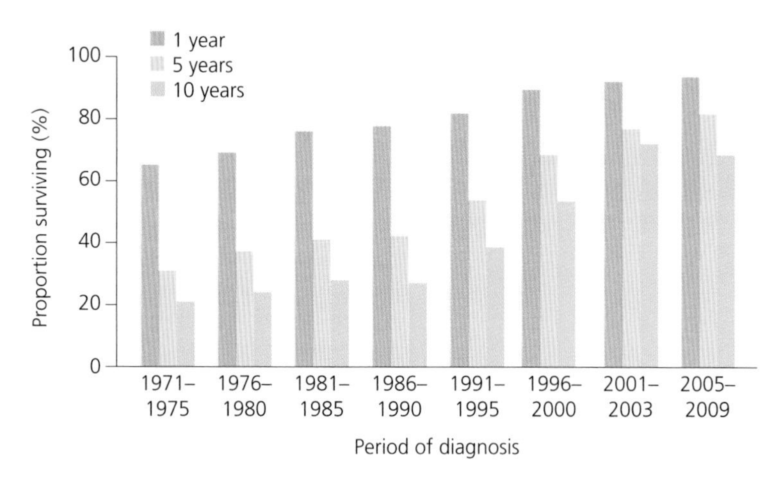

Figure 3.1 Relative survival (%) at 1, 5 and 10 years after diagnosis of prostate cancer in England and Wales (men diagnosed in eight 5-year periods from 1971 to 2009 [1- and 5-year survival] and from 1971 to predicted 2007 [10-year survival]). From 1996, 1- and 5-year data are for England only; 10-year data for 1996 to 2003 are for England only, but the 2007 predicted value is for England and Wales. Reproduced from Cancer Research UK. www.cancerresearchuk.org/cancer-info/cancerstats/survival/common-cancers.

Early detection

In general, the earlier prostate cancer is detected, the better the outlook for the patient in terms of cure or arresting cancer progression. However, we always need to be cognizant of the risk of over-diagnosis and potential over-treatment. Most patients in whom prostate cancer is suspected are identified on the basis of abnormal findings on digital rectal examination (DRE) or, more commonly now, by raised levels of PSA. An increasing majority of patients present simply with an isolated increase in PSA.

Digital rectal examination is the simplest, safest and most cost-effective means of detecting prostate cancer, provided that the tumor is posteriorly situated and is sufficiently large to be palpable. The test can be performed with the patient either in the left lateral position or standing and leaning forwards; with either approach only the posterior portion of the gland is palpable (Figure 3.2). In addition to providing information on the size of the prostate, DRE can reveal a number of features that may indicate prostate cancer (Table 3.1). However, only around one-third of suspicious prostatic nodules are actually confirmed as malignant when analyzed histologically after either transrectal or transperineal biopsy (Table 3.2).

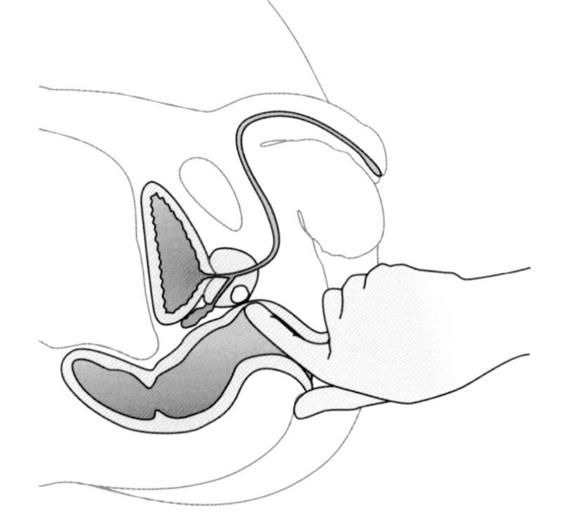

Figure 3.2 Digital rectal examination is an essential clinical test in the detection and diagnosis of prostate cancer.

TABLE 3.1

DRE findings that may indicate prostate cancer

- A nodule within one or both lobes of the gland
- Induration of part or all of the prostate
- Asymmetry of the gland
- Lack of mobility due to adhesion to surrounding tissue
- Palpable seminal vesicles

TABLE 3.2

Other causes of DRE abnormalities

- Benign prostatic hyperplasia
- Prostatic calculi
- Prostatitis (particularly granulomatous prostatitis)
- Ejaculatory duct abnormalities
- Seminal vesicle abnormalities
- Rectal mucosal polyp or tumor

Prostate-specific antigen is a glycoprotein responsible for liquefying semen. In prostatic disease, the tissue barriers become compromised, allowing PSA to enter the bloodstream (Figure 3.3). The PSA measurement in the serum is still the most effective single screening test for early detection of prostate cancer; in fact, it can detect more than twice as many prostate cancers as DRE. However, the predictive value is increased further if the measurement is combined, as it always should be, with DRE. PSA determination may also be useful in staging prostate cancer and it has especial value in evaluating the response to therapy (see Chapter 4).

Approximately 25% of men with PSA levels above 4 ng/mL have prostate cancer, and the risk increases to more than 60% in men with PSA levels above 10 ng/mL. Causes of PSA elevation in the absence of

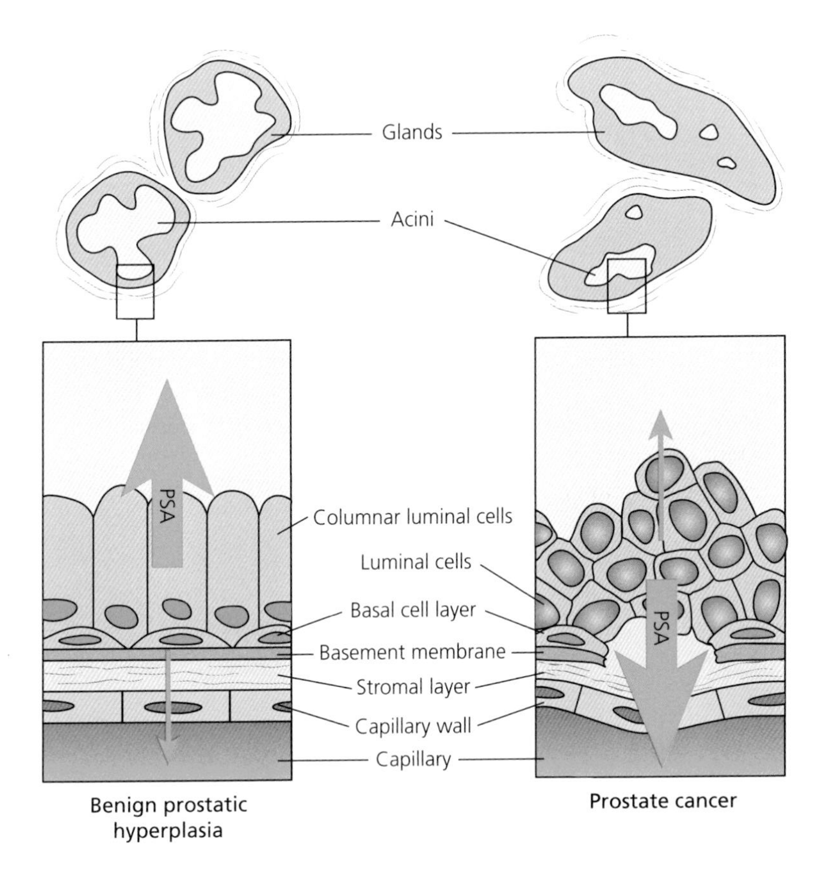

Figure 3.3 Normally, there are significant tissue barriers between the lumen of the prostate gland and the capillary bed. In prostatic diseases, especially cancer, these barriers are compromised, and serum PSA values rise.

prostate cancer are given in Table 3.3. A study in prostate cancer prevention, where all men in the placebo group received a biopsy, reported that the incidence of prostate cancer in men with PSA between 0.5 ng/mL and 4 ng/mL, and with normal DRE, was high (Table 3.4). The median PSA and 95th percentile values for the 'normal' population at each age group have been determined and are given in Table 3.5. As shown by the data in Table 3.4, a significant percentage of men with PSA values below the 95th percentile will harbor prostate cancer. There is no clear agreement on the best PSA

TABLE 3.3

Causes of PSA elevation

Prostate cancer	Perineal or prostatic trauma
Benign prostatic hyperplasia	Recent ejaculation
Prostatitis	Cycling
Urinary tract infection	

TABLE 3.4

Likelihood of prostate cancer on biopsy in men with normal DRE

PSA value (ng/mL)	Risk of prostate cancer on biopsy (%)
< 0.5	6.6
0.5–1.0	10.1
1.1–2.0	17.0
2.1–3.0	23.9
3.1–4.0	26.9

Source of data: Thompson et al., 2004.

cut-off at which men should be biopsied. In the past a cut-off of 4.0 ng/mL has been used, but a cut-off at 2.5 ng/mL would double the cancer detection rate from 18% to 36% in men younger than 60 years, and would have a minimal negative effect on specificity.

Many men with mildly elevated PSA values have benign prostatic hyperplasia (BPH) rather than prostate cancer, so it is clear that PSA is by no means a perfect test. Several different concepts have been developed over the past few years to improve the clinical value of the test in detecting early prostate cancer. These so-called PSA derivatives include PSA density, PSA velocity, age-specific reference ranges and differential assay of the different molecular forms of serum PSA. All of these have been proposed in an attempt to enhance the utility of PSA with regard to detecting early prostate cancer at a curable stage and to reduce the number of negative transrectal biopsies. In practical terms,

TABLE 3.5

Median and 95th percentile ranges of PSA in a male population

Age range (years)	Median PSA (ng/mL)	95th percentile
40–49	0.7	2.5
50–59	0.9	3.5
60–69	1.3	4.5
70–79	1.8	6.5

only the molecular forms (free:total PSA ratio) and the PSA velocity calculation are of much clinical use, as they can help the physician and patient decide whether and when to proceed to a transrectal or transperineal biopsy.

PSA density is calculated by dividing the total PSA by the prostate volume. A PSA density above 0.15 ng/mL has been shown to increase the specificity of the PSA test. This modification does, however, have many potential sources of error, such as volume calculation, assay variability and sampling bias (Figure 3.4).

PSA velocity refers to the rate of PSA change with time, usually over 1 or 2 years, with a minimum of three readings. A velocity above 0.75 ng/mL/year has been used to predict the presence of prostate cancer. More recent studies have shown that the average PSA velocity of men without prostate cancer is 0.03 ng/mL/year, compared with 0.4 ng/mL/year in men ultimately diagnosed with prostate cancer. Most recommend a PSA velocity of 0.35–0.4 ng/mL/year as a threshold to recommend biopsy, even if the PSA is within the normal range. Problems associated with PSA velocity include inaccuracy of velocity calculation over short time periods and too few measurements being made (PSA levels show natural fluctuation).

Age-specific reference ranges are predicated on the fact that the serum PSA concentration increases with age. As a result, the reference range is corrected for the patient's age (see Table 3.5). This practice increases positive-predictive values from 37% to 42%, but decreases cancer detection when compared with a cut-off of 4.0 ng/mL. Studies

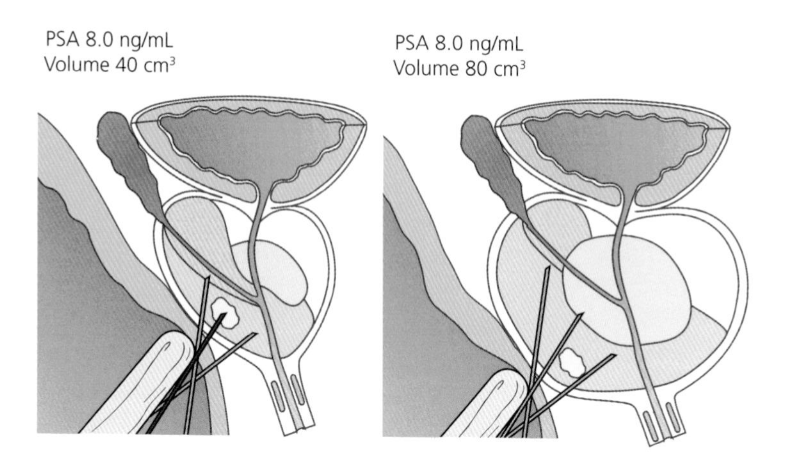

Figure 3.4 Biopsies taken from a larger prostate with a lower PSA density are less likely to sample the cancer than those taken from a smaller prostate with a higher PSA density.

have shown that age-specific median PSA values may be more useful than age-specific cut-offs, as young patients with a PSA above their age-specific median value but below a biopsy threshold of 2.5 ng/mL have an 8–14-fold increase in the risk of developing prostate cancer. Figure 3.5 shows the problem with using an age-specific cut-off rather than a standard cut-off for all ages – too many cancers are missed in older men (in whom the prevalence is greater).

Molecular forms. PSA exists in the serum in several molecular forms; most of it is bound to protein, but some is unbound or 'free'. Studies show that patients with BPH but not prostate cancer have a higher amount of free PSA, while men with prostate cancer appear to have a greater amount of PSA complexed with α_1-antichymotrypsin. Measuring the concentration of these different molecular forms in the serum is a clinically useful way to distinguish men who have BPH from men with early prostate cancer. The currently accepted cut-off point of free:total PSA is 0.15. Men with ratios below this should be considered for further investigation, including MRI and/or transrectal or transperineal prostatic biopsy.

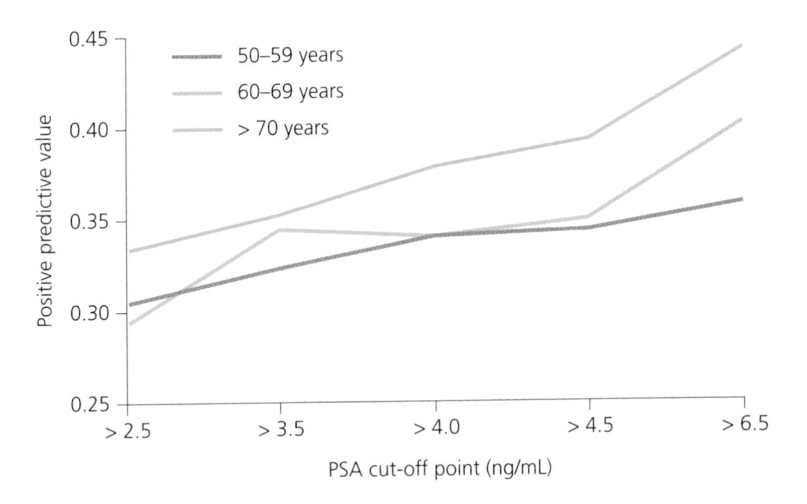

Figure 3.5 At any given PSA cut-off point the positive predictive value for older men is higher than for younger men, because of the increased prevalence of prostate cancer with age. Although raising the PSA cut-off point will increase the positive-predictive value further for older men, a proportion of men will have false-negative tests and the overall detection rate will be reduced.

Screening

The value of PSA screening asymptomatic men for prostate cancer is still highly controversial (Table 3.6). As described in Chapter 1, there is a great discrepancy between the incidence of clinically significant disease and the prevalence of microscopic disease, and identification of those men in whom disease progression is probable remains inexact.

Current evidence to support PSA screening is as follows.

- Non-randomized data show that since the advent of PSA screening in the USA and Europe, the proportion of men presenting with advanced prostate cancer has decreased, as has prostate cancer mortality.
- In one randomized study, men with clinically significant prostate cancer treated with radical prostatectomy had a 44% reduction in risk of premature death compared with conservative management.
- The PSA test and DRE are simple to perform and the prostate biopsy has a relatively low complication rate (around 2–4%).

TABLE 3.6

Screening for prostate cancer

Pros

- Simple tests available (PSA and DRE)
- Detects early, potentially curable lesions
- Reassures those who are screened as negative
- Screening reduces mortality by up to 56%

Cons

- False-positive findings cause anxiety
- Biopsy guided by transrectal ultrasonography carries a 2% risk of serious infective complications and causes anxiety
- Expensive
- Some small slow-growing cancers will be treated unnecessarily, and treatment has side effects

Disadvantages to screening include the following.

- There is a potential to detect and treat clinically insignificant cancers that may be better left undetected.
- The PIVOT trial showed little benefit of surgery compared with watchful waiting in men with lower-risk cancers.
- There is a significant morbidity associated with prostate cancer diagnosis and treatment.
- A large proportion of men having a biopsy will not harbor prostate cancer, and biopsies have an associated morbidity.
- The screening process may generate anxiety.

The most recent American Urological Association (AUA) guidelines recommend against PSA screening in men under 40 years of age and do not recommend routine screening in men aged 40–54 years and judged to be at average risk, as men of this age were not included in the randomized screening studies. For those men younger than 55 but with risk factors for prostate cancer (see page 8), decisions about screening should be individualized. The strongest evidence for a benefit of screening is in men aged 55 to 69 years; the AUA guidelines recommend that decisions about screening for men aged 55–69 should be shared between the man and his clinician, and based on the individual's values and preferences.

Early results from two large randomized studies and longer-term results from a third randomized study have been reported. The larger European study (the European Randomized Study of Screening for Prostate Cancer [ERSPC]) randomized men to screening at 4-yearly intervals or no screening. A biopsy was mandated if the PSA was above 3.0 ng/mL or an abnormal DRE was detected. This study reported a 27% reduction in prostate cancer mortality at a median follow-up of 9 years. Unfortunately, the number of men needed to treat to save one man from death was 48. A report on a subset of men in this trial from Gothenburg, Sweden, with a median 14-year follow-up, showed a higher cumulative incidence of prostate cancer among the screened population (Figure 3.6). Prostate cancer mortality was reduced by 44% in those randomized to screening. In men who actually attended screening, prostate cancer mortality was reduced by 56%. With longer follow-up, the number needed to treat to save one man was reduced to 12.

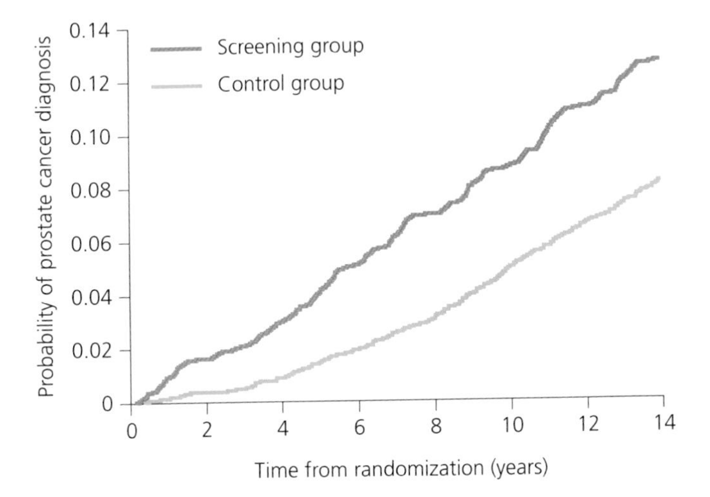

Figure 3.6 Cumulative incidence of prostate cancer in men randomized to screening or observation in the Göteborg Randomised Population-based Prostate-cancer Screening Trial. Reproduced with permission from Hugosson et al. *Lancet Oncol* 2010;11:725–32.

In contrast, the smaller US study (the Prostate, Lung, Colorectal, and Ovarian [PLCO] Cancer Screening Trial) failed to report a mortality benefit at a shorter follow-up, although this trial was somewhat flawed by excessive PSA screening in the control arm.

A recently updated Cochrane meta-analysis of five randomized controlled trials concluded that screening did not result in a statistically significant reduction in prostate cancer-specific mortality when all populations of all studies were included (risk ratio 1.0 [0.86–1.17]) (Figure 3.7). Currently, the US Preventive Services Task Force advises against PSA screening in all men.

In the future, it seems likely that screening will be focused on men who are genetically most susceptible to prostate cancer. More than 70 'prostate cancer susceptibility genes' have been discovered. Men with mutations of these could be targeted for screening.

Right now, the family physician has an important role in assessing the likely benefits and risks for individual patients according to their age and life expectancy; appropriate counseling of the patient and his immediate family is an essential element of this process.

Men with a PSA above the median for their age (see Table 3.5) should be recognized as having a higher risk for prostate cancer. Patients with an

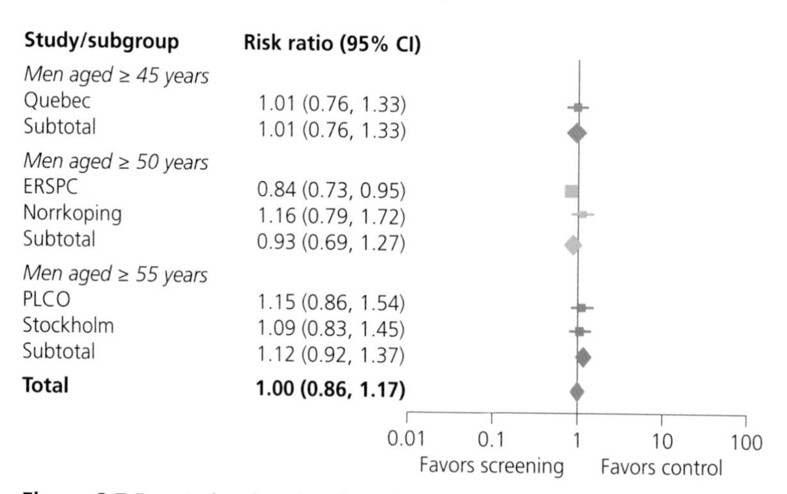

Figure 3.7 Forest plot showing the risk ratios for prostate-cancer mortality in men screened for the disease versus controls: a meta-analysis of five randomized trials. Adapted from Ilic D et al. 2013.

abnormal screening test, either from DRE or age-specific PSA, or an abnormal increase in PSA from a previous result (PSA velocity) should be referred to a urologist. The decision to biopsy will be based not simply on a single PSA value but on a patient's risk factors, including: race and family history; previous PSA values; previous biopsy results; and assessment of comorbidities and life expectancy. The patient's own preferences should be central in the decision-making process.

Clinical symptoms

Patients with prostate cancer may present with a variety of symptoms (Table 3.7), some of which overlap with those of BPH.

Localized cancer is generally asymptomatic. Men will most often present with symptoms of BPH that are unrelated to the cancer. These symptoms occur when benign prostatic tissue compresses and obstructs the urethra, resulting in frequency, hesitancy and poor flow.

TABLE 3.7

Clinical presentation/symptoms of local and locally invasive prostate cancer

Local disease	Locally invasive disease
• Asymptomatic	• Hematuria
• Elevated PSA	• Dysuria
• BPH symptoms	• Perineal and suprapubic pain
– weak stream	• Erectile dysfunction
– hesitancy	• Incontinence
– sensation of incomplete emptying	• Loin pain or anuria resulting from obstruction of the ureters
– frequency	• Symptoms of renal failure
– urgency	• Hemospermia
– urge incontinence	• Rectal symptoms, including tenesmus
– urinary tract infection	

BPH, benign prostatic hyperplasia; PSA, prostate-specific antigen.

Prostate cancer may also present as an 'incidental' finding after TURP (Figure 3.8); nowadays, fewer than 10% of men undergoing TURP for BPH are found to have microscopic foci of prostate cancer.

Locally advanced cancers (usually palpable by DRE) may cause symptoms resulting from local extension of the tumor, such as irritative symptoms (frequency, urgency) that can occur as a result of invasion of the bladder trigone and pelvic nerves. Involvement of the perineal or suprapubic nerves can lead to pain, and thus the possibility of prostate cancer should be considered in the investigation of prostatitis-like symptoms.

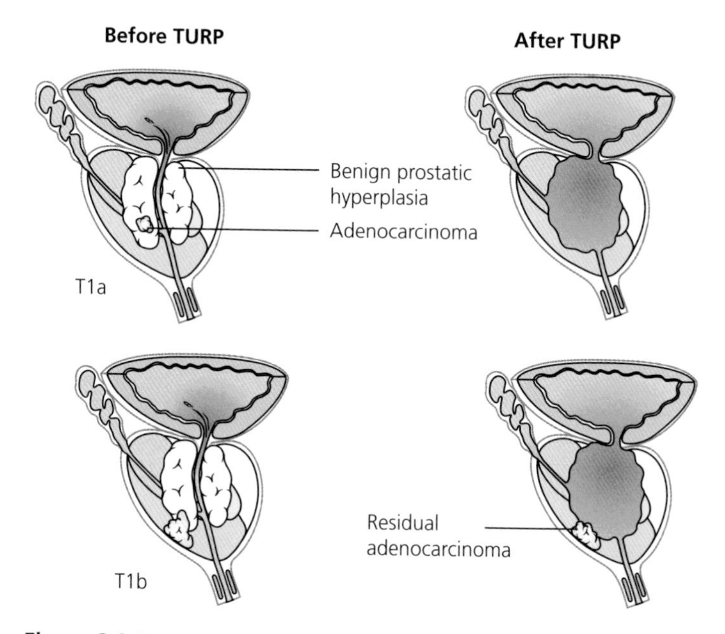

Figure 3.8 Prostate cancer is found in resected chips of prostate tissue obtained during transurethral resection of the prostate (TURP) in up to 10% of cases. About two-thirds of the cancers are well-differentiated T1a lesions involving less than 5% of the chips. The remaining lesions are T1b cancers that have larger volume and are less well differentiated. A number of potential sampling errors are inherent in the diagnosis of prostate cancer at TURP. T1a tumors that are confined to the transition zone may be completely excised, whereas significant amounts of T1b tumors may remain after the procedure.

Hematuria can occur from local spread of the cancer into the urethra or bladder. Loin pain can occur because of ureteric obstruction and hydronephrosis. Symptoms of bladder outlet obstruction can occur when a large cancer obstructs the bladder outlet, similar to BPH. Invasion of the urethral sphincter or, more commonly, surgery itself may cause urinary incontinence. It is important to exclude the possibility that incontinence is a result of chronic urinary retention with overflow, which may be treatable with procedures such as TURP. Constipation, tenesmus and rectal bleeding can result from the large prostate distorting the rectum. Invasion of the seminal vesicles may occasionally result in hemospermia, but this is not a common presenting symptom.

Metastatic disease. The most common presenting symptoms are shown in Table 3.8. Pain resulting from bony metastases, particularly in the pelvis and lumbar spine, is the major symptom; thus, the sudden onset of progressive low back or pelvic pain is an important diagnostic feature of metastatic prostate cancer. Pathological fractures may also occur, particularly affecting the neck of the femur. Metastases within the vertebrae, sometimes leading to spinal cord compression, are not uncommon and may produce backache or neurological symptoms in up to 12% of affected men.

TABLE 3.8

Presenting symptoms of metastatic prostate cancer

Distant metastases

- Bone pain or sciatica
- Paraplegia secondary to spinal cord compression
- Lymph node enlargement
- Loin pain or anuria due to obstruction of ureters by lymph nodes

Widespread metastases

- Lethargy (from anemia or uremia, for example)
- Weight loss and cachexia
- Cutaneous and bowel hemorrhage (unusual)

Metastasis into the lymph nodes may result in lymph node enlargement. Intra-abdominal lymph node metastasis usually begins in the obturator and internal iliac nodes, spreads to the iliac nodes and beyond and may, with local tumors, result in obstruction of the ureters. In advanced disease, lymphatic involvement may extend to the thoracic, cervical, inguinal and axillary nodes. Lymph node metastases may produce a number of symptoms, including palpable swellings, loin pain or anuria due to obstruction of the ureters, and swelling of the lower limbs as a result of lymphedema.

Systemic metastases in the liver, lungs or elsewhere may produce non-specific symptoms, such as lethargy resulting from anemia or uremia, weight loss and cachexia.

Key points – screening and early detection

- Increasingly, prostate cancer is being diagnosed on the basis of a raised level of prostate-specific antigen (PSA) and subsequent investigation.
- PSA-based screening of asymptomatic men is controversial.
- Transrectal ultrasound-guided biopsies are needed to confirm the diagnosis.
- More advanced disease can present with symptoms of bladder outflow obstruction.
- Bone metastases may cause bone pain or pathological fracture.

Key references

Andriole GL, Bostwick DG, Brawley OW et al. Effect of dutasteride on the risk of prostate cancer. *N Engl J Med* 2010;362:1192–202.

Brooks JD, Metter EJ, Chan DW et al. Plasma selenium level before diagnosis and the risk of prostate cancer development. *J Urol* 2001;166:2034–8.

Carter BH, Albertsen PC, Barry MJ et al. American Urologic Association. Early detection of prostate cancer: AUA Guideline 2013. Available from www.auanet.org/common/pdf/education/clinical-guidance/Prostate-Cancer-Detection.pdf, last accessed 01 November 2013.

Cohen YC, Liu KS, Heyden NL et al. Detection bias due to the effect of finasteride on prostate volume: a modeling approach for analysis of the Prostate Cancer Prevention Trial. *J Natl Cancer Inst* 2007;99:1366–74.

Duffield-Lillico AJ, Dalkin BL, Reid ME et al. Selenium supplementation, baseline plasma selenium status and incidence of prostate cancer: an analysis of the complete treatment period of the Nutritional Prevention of Cancer Trial. *BJU Int* 2003;91:608–12.

Giovannucci E, Liu Y, Platz EA et al. Risk factors for prostate cancer incidence and progression in the health professionals follow-up study. *Int J Cancer* 2007;121:1571–8.

Gomella L. Chemoprevention using dutasteride: the REDUCE trial. *Curr Opin Urol* 2005;15:29–32.

Ilic D, Neuberger MM, Djulbegovic M, Dahm P. Screening for prostate cancer (review). *Cochrane Database Syst Rev* 2013;(1):CD004720.

Lippmani SM, Klein EA, Goodman PJ et al. Effect of selenium and vitamin E on risk of prostate cancer and other cancers: the Selenium and Vitamin E Cancer Prevention Trial (SELECT). *JAMA* 2009;301:39–51.

Lucia MS, Epstein JI, Goodman PJ et al. Finasteride and high-grade prostate cancer in the Prostate Cancer Prevention Trial. *J Natl Cancer Inst* 2007;99:1375–83.

Miller EC, Giovannucci E, Erdman JW Jr et al. Tomato products, lycopene, and prostate cancer risk. *Urol Clin North Am* 2002;29:83–93.

Shepherd BE, Redman MW, Ankerst DP. Does finasteride affect the severity of prostate cancer? A causal sensitivity analysis. *J Am Stat Assoc* 2008;103:1392–404.

Thompson IM, Chi C, Ankerst DP et al. Effect of finasteride on the sensitivity of PSA for detecting prostate cancer. *J Natl Cancer Inst* 2006;98:1128–33.

Thompson IM, Goodman PJ, Tangen CM et al. The influence of finasteride on the development of prostate cancer. *N Engl J Med* 2003;349:215–24.

Thompson IM, Pauler DK, Goodman PJ et al. Prevalence of prostate cancer among men with a prostate-specific antigen level < or =4.0 ng per milliliter. *N Engl J Med* 2004;350:2239–46.

US Preventive Services Task Force. *Recommendation Statement: Screening for Prostate Cancer.* www.uspreventiveservicestaskforce.org/prostatecancerscreening/prostatefinalrs.htm, last accessed 30 October 2013.

Vickers AJ, Ulmert D, Sjoberg DD et al. Strategy for detection of prostate cancer based on relation between prostate specific antigen at age 40–55 and long term risk of metastasis: case-control study. *BMJ* 2013;346:f2023.

Virtamo J, Pietinen P, Huttunen JK et al. Incidence of cancer and mortality following alpha-tocopherol and beta-carotene supplementation: a postintervention follow-up. *JAMA* 2003;290:476–85.

4 Prognostic indicators and staging

Accurate grading and staging of prostate cancer, particularly distinguishing between Gleason grades and between localized and more extensive disease, is critical for selection of the optimum treatment option. Although developments in imaging techniques, especially MRI, have led to more accurate staging than can be achieved with digital rectal examination (DRE) or prostate-specific antigen (PSA) testing alone, both under- and overstaging are still common clinical problems. Thus, a need remains not only for improved staging techniques, but also for better prognostic markers that will give an indication of future disease behavior if left untreated.

Staging of localized disease

Staging of localized disease relies primarily on the following techniques:

- DRE
- PSA measurement
- transrectal ultrasonography (TRUS) and ultrasound-guided biopsy
- CT scanning
- MRI – using multiparametric technology
- bone scanning
- choline positron emission tomography (PET)/CT scanning
- tables and nomograms to predict disease stage and outcome.

Digital rectal examination. Accuracy in staging prostate cancer by DRE is only 30–50%; underestimation is common because small and anteriorly located tumors are generally impalpable, and false-positive findings may occur in patients with conditions such as benign prostatic hyperplasia (BPH) or prostatitis. The technique can, however, detect a number of significant cancers when PSA is still within the normal range (< 4.0 ng/mL) and provide useful, if imprecise, information about the local stage of the disease (see Chapter 1).

Prostate-specific antigen determination. Within overall groups of patients, there is a reasonable correlation between PSA levels and the clinical stage (and, to a lesser extent, the pathological stage) of prostate cancer. The correlation is poorer, however, in individual patients because of the considerable overlap between the PSA ranges associated with different stages. PSA levels above 20 ng/mL are often indicative of tumor extension beyond the prostatic capsule, while levels above 40 ng/mL suggest a high likelihood of bony or soft tissue metastases (see the Memorial Sloan-Kettering Cancer Center's pretreatment nomogram at http://nomograms.mskcc.org/Prostate/PreTreatment.aspx). Figure 4.1 shows the relationship between PSA level before radical prostatectomy and likelihood of PSA-free progression.

PSA velocity has also been shown to be helpful in identifying men with more aggressive disease in some studies. A study from the USA observed that men who had a velocity above 2.0 ng/mL/year immediately before diagnosis were at high risk of death from prostate cancer, irrespective of treatment.

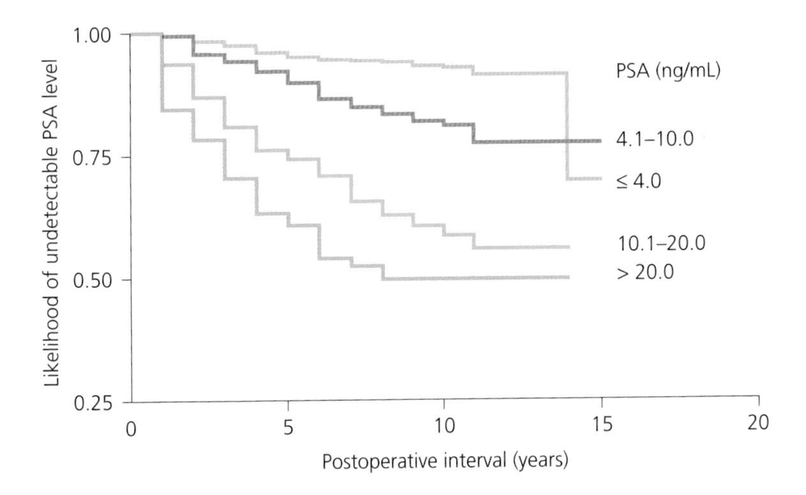

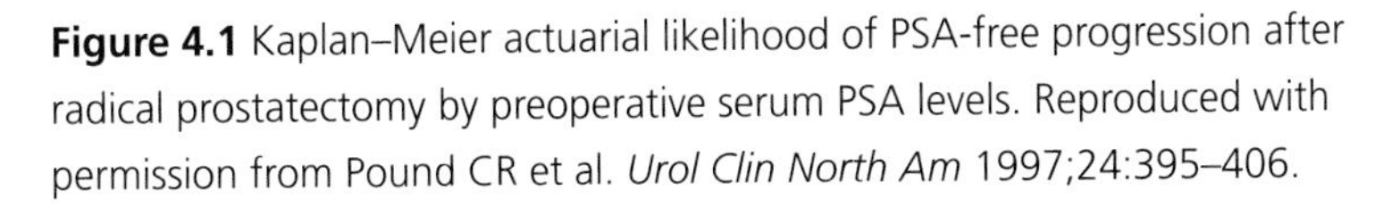
Figure 4.1 Kaplan–Meier actuarial likelihood of PSA-free progression after radical prostatectomy by preoperative serum PSA levels. Reproduced with permission from Pound CR et al. *Urol Clin North Am* 1997;24:395–406.

Although the serum PSA concentration alone may not be a precise indicator of stage on an individual basis, it can sometimes be used to eliminate some staging investigations. It appears that men who present with newly diagnosed well- or moderately well-differentiated prostate cancer, no skeletal symptoms and a serum PSA value less than or equal to 10 ng/mL may not always need a staging radionuclide bone scan. For these individuals, the probability of having skeletal metastases approaches zero. Many clinicians, however, still like to use this test as a baseline investigation because it may identify 'hot spots' due to conditions such as degenerative osteoarthritis that may cause confusion later – if or when the PSA level starts to rise. A negative scan also serves to reassure a patient that his skeleton is not involved.

Transrectal ultrasonography has a number of uses in the management of prostate cancer. It is most commonly used to image the prostate gland and direct the biopsy sampling device to the appropriate spot during prostate biopsy (Figure 4.2). Antibiotics are obligatory before

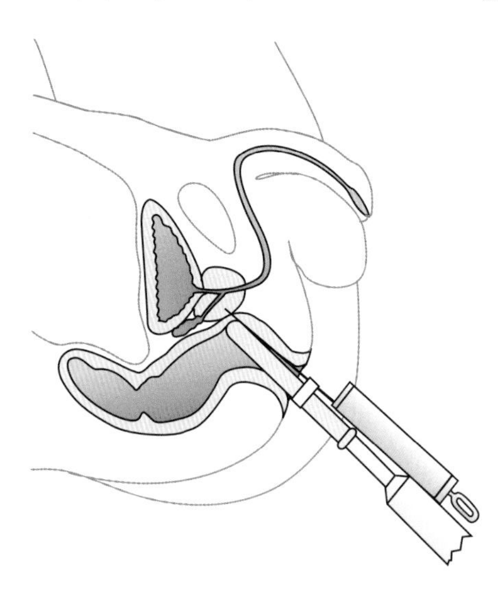

Figure 4.2 Transrectal ultrasonography (TRUS)-guided biopsy. An ultrasound probe is introduced into the rectum to lie adjacent to the prostate. Under antibiotic cover and ultrasound control, multiple prostatic biopsies may be taken with an automatic biopsy gun.

and after the procedure to reduce the risk of infection, currently estimated at around 2%, although this may be rising because of the increases in the antibiotic resistance of bacteria, particularly *Escherichia coli*. A quinolone is the usual choice, sometimes in combination with gentamicin or amikacin, depending on prostate size, personal preference and previous biopsy results. Usually 8–14 TRUS-guided biopsies are taken from different regions of the prostate with an 18-gauge needle. This is now routinely performed on an outpatient basis, after infiltration with local anesthesia. The percentage of each biopsy core involved and the overall number of positive biopsy specimens provide a useful estimate of tumor volume (Figure 4.3). In high-risk cases (large bulky palpable tumors, or PSA > 20 ng/mL), additional lateral capsular and seminal vesicle biopsies can be taken with minimal extra morbidity to confirm or exclude extraprostatic extension. Transperineal template biopsies under general anesthesia allow extended sampling of the gland, but with an increased risk of urinary retention. Because of the much lower risk of infection, many urologists are employing transperineal template biopsies in preference to the transrectal type.

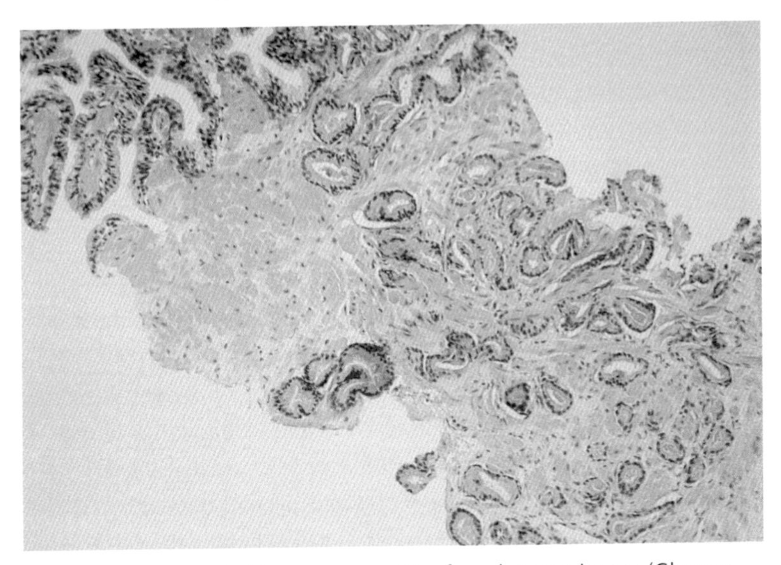

Figure 4.3 A prostatic biopsy core positive for adenocarcinoma (Gleason grades 3 and 4, Gleason score 7).

Cancer within the prostate gland is not reliably apparent ultrasonographically, but occasionally can present with a number of ultrasonographic abnormalities. These include abnormal echo patterns (usually hypoechoic); loss of differentiation between central and peripheral zones; asymmetry of size or shape; and capsular distortion.

Some prostate tumors are hypoechoic, but hypoechoic images may result from other causes, so the specificity of this finding for prostate cancer is only 20–25%. Assessment of local staging by TRUS imaging alone is poor. When extracapsular extension or seminal vesicle extension is suspected on imaging, a biopsy of the suspicious area is required for confirmation.

***PCA3* (Prostate CAncer gene 3)** is a piece of non-coding RNA that is only present in the prostate. It has value as a biomarker because levels in prostate cancer tissue are greatly increased (up to 66-fold). In contrast, it is not increased in benign conditions such as BPH. The *PCA3* test also appears to be sensitive, detecting increases in tissue samples containing fewer than 10% cancer cells. *PCA3* score is positively associated with the probability of a positive biopsy, and the relationship appears to be unaffected by prostate volume, prostatitis, number of prior biopsies or 5α-reductase inhibitor treatment for BPH. *PCA3* is becoming incorporated into diagnostic nomograms, and research is continuing into its role in prostate cancer prediction and monitoring. It seems likely that the major value of the *PCA3* test will be to reduce the number of repeat biopsies.

Prolaris is a genomic 'risk stratification' test that can add prognostic information to a patient's picture. It quantitatively measures the RNA expression levels of 31 genes involved in tumor cell division plus 15 'housekeeper' genes that allow standardization of the test. Low levels of expression of these genes is associated with low risk of cancer progression and vice versa. The manufacturers claim that the test can identify low- and intermediate-risk patients and those who are potentially at higher risk. Several clinical trials support the value of Prolaris, and further studies are under way.

Other companies are producing similar genomic prognostic tests; for example, the Oncotype DX prostate cancer assay. Studies to confirm the effectiveness of this assay are under way.

Computerized tomography has virtually no role in the local staging of prostate cancer, as separation from surrounding muscle is poor and intraprostatic anatomy is not well defined. Its primary role is in the detection of nodal and other soft tissue metastases. The sensitivity of this modality is around 36%, because the criterion for detection of positive disease is based on nodal size (> 10 mm) and CT is not able to detect microscopic nodal metastases, which are much more common. Although CT can be used to monitor bone metastases, bone scans, ^{11}C-choline PET/CT and MRI are far superior.

Magnetic resonance imaging

Multiparametric MRI is increasingly used to identify 'areas of interest', so that biopsies can be better targeted, and to stage prostate cancer. It gives excellent zonal anatomy and prostate cancer can be identified as a hypodense lesion on T2-weighted images (Figure 4.4).

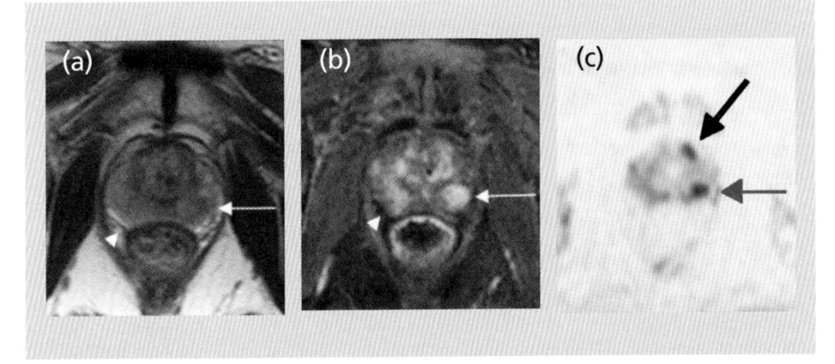

Figure 4.4 MRI scans of a prostate gland: (a) shows suspicious areas in the left (arrow) and right (arrow head) peripheral zone on T2-weighted imaging; (b) dynamic contrast enhancement shows early contrast enhancement of the left peripheral zone lesion (arrow); (c) a diffusion-weighted image highlights the left peripheral zone lesion (red arrow) as well as a left anterior lesion (black arrow). Reproduced with permission from Iwazawa J et al. *Diagn Interv Radiol* 2011;17:243–8.

It is more difficult to identify on T2-weighted images in the transition zone. Identification of extracapsular extension or invasion into the seminal vesicles depends on identification of hypodense regions in the normally bright periprostatic fat or seminal vesicles. It may, however, depend on more subtle changes such as asymmetry of the neurovascular bundles, irregular gland margins or capsular obliteration. The sensitivity of MRI for the detection of extracapsular extension has been reported to range from 13% to 95%, and accuracy is certainly higher in those units with a lot of experience in interpreting prostate images. MRI has little advantage over CT in the evaluation of nodal metastases. However, promising results have been reported with the use of ultrasmall superparamagnetic iron oxide particles as an aid to nodal metastasis evaluation by MRI.

Magnetic resonance spectroscopy. The addition of magnetic resonance (MR) spectroscopy (i.e. evaluating chemical metabolites in a small volume of interest using MR technology) has also improved the accuracy of MR staging.

Dynamic contrast-enhanced MRI is a method of imaging the prostate during rapid infusion of gadolinium contrast. Prostate cancer is detected based on early enhancement and early wash-out resulting from angiogenesis. While this enhancement is typical, it is not specific and has a sensitivity of 46–96% and specificity of 74–96% for defining prostate cancer.

Diffusion-weighted MRI generates maps of diffusion of water within tissues and uses the fact that water diffuses more easily in normal prostate (loosely packed glands) than prostate cancer (tightly packed glands). This modality can also be used to gain an impression of the aggressiveness of the cancer, as highly aggressive tumors show poorer diffusion of water. Sensitivities and specificities for the detection of prostate cancer are reported to be 57–93.3% and 57–100%, respectively. The combination of all four MRI methods significantly improves the detection and local staging of prostate cancer by MRI. It is increasingly used before prostate biopsy to target suspicious areas and to follow up patients managed by active surveillance. Some are now arguing that it is a prerequisite ahead of biopsy to improve the accuracy of the technique.

Positron emission tomography is a functional imaging technique that uses specific molecular probes labeled with radionuclides. ^{18}F-FDG is widely used for other cancers, but the results are mixed for prostate cancer. This has led to the investigation of other tracers, such as ^{11}C-acetate, ^{11}C-choline and ^{18}F-choline in recent years. ^{11}C-choline PET combined with CT appears particularly useful for staging high-risk prostate cancer (Figure 4.5). A study comparing the sensitivities and specificities of MRI, ^{11}C-choline PET and ^{11}C-choline PET/CT for the detection of nodal disease in men with high-risk localized prostate cancer found ^{11}C-choline PET/CT to be the most accurate method (Table 4.1).

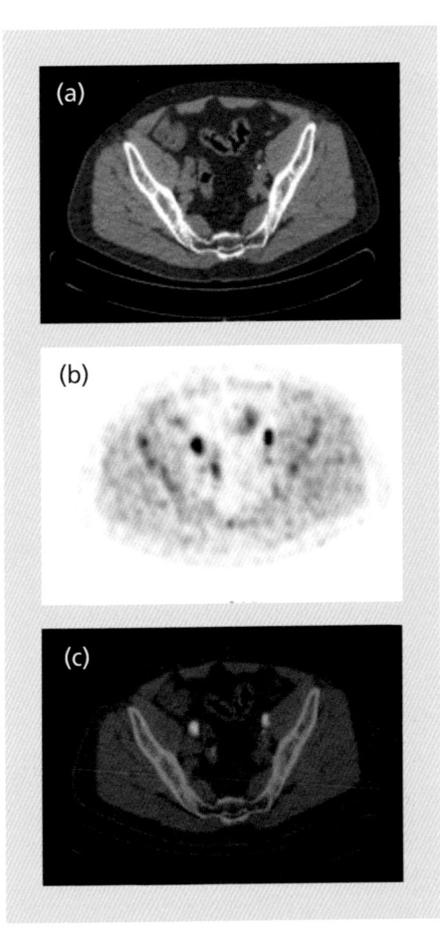

Figure 4.5 Images from a patient, 71 years, with biopsy-proven prostate cancer. ^{18}F-choline PET/CT staging showed advanced disease (iliacal lymph node metastases shown here). (a) CT scan, (b) PET scan and (c) PET/CT fused image. Reproduced with permission from Schwarzenböck S et al. *Theranostics* 2012; 2:318–330.

TABLE 4.1

Diagnostic performance for assessing lymph node status in men with high-risk localized prostate cancer

Diagnostic indicator (per patient)	MRI	^{11}C-choline PET	^{11}C-choline PET/CT
Sensitivity (%)	50.0	66.7	77.8
Specificity (%)	72.2	76.4	82.4

Data from Contractor K et al. *Clin Cancer Res* 2011;17:7673.

Prognostic tables and nomograms. While cancer characteristics such as PSA, Gleason score, clinical stage, number of biopsy cores involved and percentage of each core involved provide valuable prognostic information, combining all of these variables in a nomogram gives a much more accurate prediction of the patient's outcome. Many of these nomograms are available on the web or for use on personal digital assistants (PDAs). See, for example, the Memorial Sloan-Kettering Cancer Center's pretreatment nomogram at http://nomograms.mskcc.org/Prostate/PreTreatment.aspx. Nomograms have been developed, based on the data from thousands of patients, that predict the pathological likelihood of seminal vesicle invasion, lymph node metastasis and extracapsular extension on each side or presence of a small, insignificant cancer. Other nomograms have been developed to predict the likelihood of recurrence of cancer after treatment by radical prostatectomy, external-beam radiotherapy and brachytherapy. More simple prediction tools, such as Partin's tables, predict the likely pathology from values of PSA, Gleason score and clinical stage. These readily available clinical predictors are very useful for patient counseling and making treatment decisions, as well as for planning treatment such as surgery or radiotherapy.

Staging of metastatic disease

This involves assessing the extent of bone and soft tissue involvement. The principal techniques used are a chest X-ray, radionuclide bone scanning, CT and MRI and, more recently, ^{11}C-choline PET/CT.

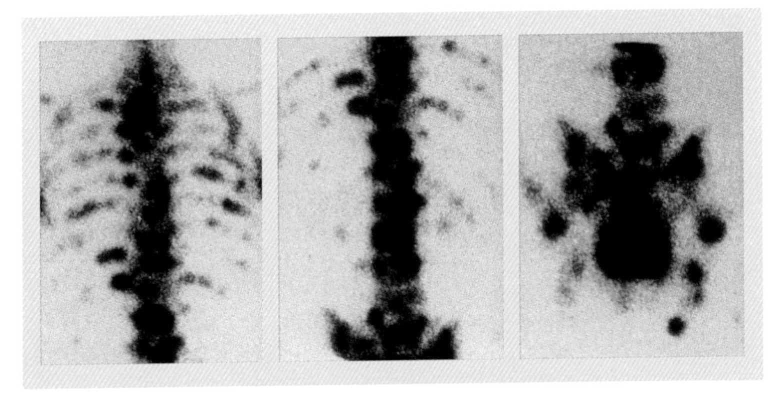

Figure 4.6 A radionuclide bone scan showing multiple bony metastases resulting from disseminated prostate cancer.

Radionuclide bone scanning is usually performed as a baseline assessment at the time of the initial diagnosis of prostate cancer (Figure 4.6). If the PSA value is less than 10 ng/mL and the Gleason score is below 8, it may be permissible to omit this test as it is so rarely positive in these circumstances. The use of this technique in routine follow-up has declined, as serial PSA measurements have been shown to be the most accurate and cost-effective means of monitoring bony metastases.

Computerized tomography of the abdomen and pelvis may be used in cases in which treatment decisions depend on the presence and degree of lymph node or other soft tissue involvement. Small-volume and microscopic metastases (< 1 cm) are not usually detectable by this technique, and thus the accuracy of CT scanning is only 40–50%. CT scanning may also be employed occasionally to guide fine needle aspiration of enlarged lymph nodes for cytological analysis to aid diagnosis.

Magnetic resonance imaging can also be used to identify metastatic disease affecting the regional lymph nodes. However, most scanners do not easily permit guided fine needle aspiration. MRI may also be useful for clarifying the nature of any abnormality in equivocal bone scans and, importantly, for recognizing incipient spinal cord compression.

Positron emission tomography/CT scanning. ^{11}C-choline PET/CT images (see page 51) are also an accurate method of staging advanced disease.

Immunoscintigraphy using radioactive antibodies directed against prostate-specific proteins has proved inadequate for clinical use in its present form owing to its lack of specificity and sensitivity.

Summary of treatment options

An approach to the diagnosis and staging of prostate cancer is outlined in Figure 4.7.

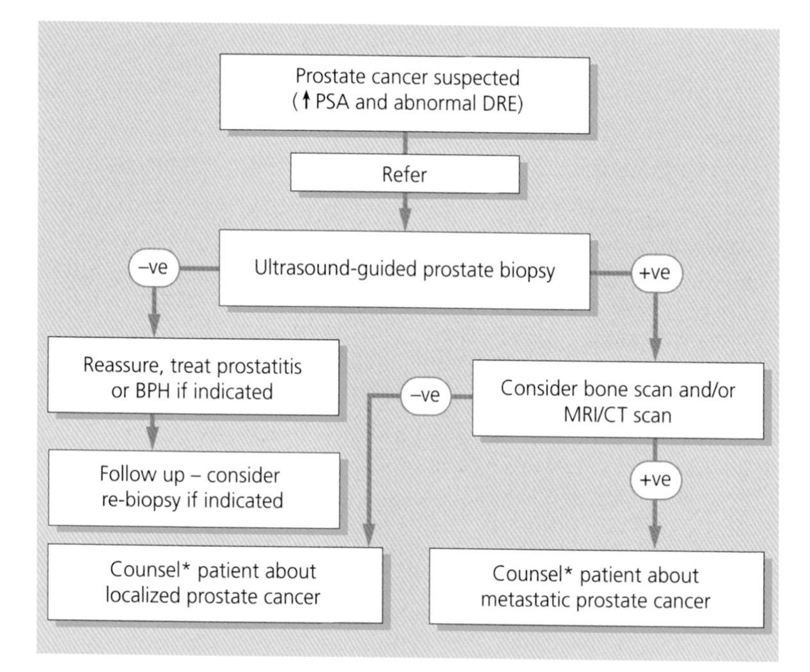

Figure 4.7 Algorithm for diagnosis and staging of prostate cancer. +ve, positive; –ve, negative; BPH, benign prostatic hyperplasia; DRE, digital rectal examination; PSA, prostate-specific antigen. *Involving the informed patient and his relatives in the decision-making process.

Key points – prognostic indicators and staging

- Prostate cancer is usually diagnosed on the basis of transrectal or transperineal biopsy under antibiotic cover and local anesthesia.
- The Gleason score of these biopsies, the clinical stage on DRE and the presenting PSA value provide an estimate of the risk of extraprostatic extension.
- MRI is increasingly used to target biopsies and can provide information about local staging.
- Bone scanning identifies bone metastases, but the probability of these with PSA < 10 ng/mL is low.
- PET/CT is also a useful way of detecting metastases.

Key references

Bouchelouche K, Turkbey B, Choyke P, Capala J. Imaging prostate cancer: an update on positron emission tomography and magnetic resonance imaging. *Curr Urol Rep* 2010;11:180–90.

Contractor K, Challapalli A, Barwick T et al. Use of [11C]choline PET-CT as a noninvasive method for detecting pelvic lymph node status from prostate cancer and relationship with choline kinase expression. *Clin Cancer Res* 2011;17:7673–83.

D'Amico AV, Chen MH, Roehl KA, Catalona WJ. Preoperative PSA velocity and the risk of death from prostate cancer after radical prostatectomy. *N Engl J Med* 2004;351:125–35.

Eifler JB, Feng Z, Lin BM et al. An updated prostate cancer staging nomogram (Partin tables) based on cases from 2006 to 2011. *BJU Int* 2013;111:22–9.

Gacci M, Schiavina R, Lanciotti M et al. External validation of the updated nomogram predicting lymph node invasion in patients with prostate cancer undergoing extended pelvic lymph node dissection. *Urol Int* 2013;90:277–82.

Harisinghani MG, Barentsz J, Hahn PF et al. Noninvasive detection of clinically occult lymph-node metastases in prostate cancer. *N Engl J Med* 2003;348:2491–9.

Hricak H, Choyke PL, Eberhardt SC et al. Imaging prostate cancer: a multidisciplinary perspective. *Radiology* 2007;243:28–53.

Ishizuka O, Tanabe T, Nakayama T et al. Prostate-specific antigen, Gleason sum and clinical T stage for predicting the need for radionuclide bone scan for prostate cancer patients in Japan. *Int J Urol* 2005;12:728–32.

Kattan MW, Eastham JA, Wheeler TM et al. Counseling men with prostate cancer: a nomogram for predicting the presence of small, moderately differentiated, confined tumors. *J Urol* 2003;170:1792–7.

Kattan MW, Zelefsky MJ, Kupelian PA et al. Pretreatment nomogram that predicts 5-year probability of metastasis following three-dimensional conformal radiation therapy for localized prostate cancer. *J Clin Oncol* 2003;21:4568–71.

Moore CM, Robertson NL, Arsanious N et al. Image-guided prostate biopsy using magnetic resonance imaging-derived targets: a systematic review. *Eur Urol* 2013;63:125–40.

Ohori M, Kattan MW, Koh H et al. Predicting the presence and side of extracapsular extension: a nomogram for staging prostate cancer. *J Urol* 2004;171:1844–9; discussion 1849.

Partin AW, Mangold LA, Lamm DM et al. Contemporary update of prostate cancer staging nomograms (Partin Tables) for the new millennium. *Urology* 2001;58: 843–8.

Pound CR, Partin AW, Epstein JI, Walsh PC. Prostate-specific antigen after anatomic radical retropubic prostatectomy. Patterns of recurrence and cancer control. *Urol Clin North Am* 1997;24:395–406.

Stephenson AJ, Kattan MW. Nomograms for prostate cancer. *BJU Int* 2006;98:39–46.

Taneja SS, Hsu EI, Cheli CD et al. Complexed prostate-specific antigen as a staging tool: results based on a multicenter prospective evaluation of complexed prostate-specific antigen in cancer diagnosis. *Urology* 2002;60(suppl 1):10–17.

Turkbey B, Choyke PL. Multiparametric MRI and prostate cancer diagnosis and risk stratification. *Curr Opin Urol* 2012;22:310–15

Wang L, Hricak H, Kattan MW et al. Prediction of organ-confined prostate cancer: incremental value of MR imaging and MR spectroscopic imaging to staging nomograms. *Radiology* 2006;238:597–603.

5 Management of localized and high-risk disease

Management of localized prostate cancer

There are a number of treatment options available for men with localized prostate cancer (Table 5.1). Treatment decisions depend on many factors; however, at the core is the risk category into which the man falls. These risk groups are generally divided into very low, low, intermediate and high-risk of recurrence and are based on Gleason score, number of biopsy cores involved, PSA level and clinical stage (Table 5.2). Unfortunately, our current knowledge is such that it is not always possible to predict which treatments will produce the optimum outcome for an individual, so patient choice is a very important factor. It may be possible to build a prognostic picture using genetic markers of cell cycle progression (CCP). Prolaris, for example, is a genomic test that measures the expression levels of genes involved with cancer replication in tumor material from biopsy (see page 48); promising results suggest it will add prognostic value to current methods. Other gene-based tests are in the pipeline.

The aim of treatment of men with localized prostate cancer of significant grade and volume is often curative if the man has a reasonable life expectancy, or prevention of death **from** prostate cancer (as opposed to death **with** prostate cancer in men with shorter anticipated life spans). The likelihood of a man with localized prostate cancer dying from prostate cancer, as opposed to other causes, increases with his risk category, but decreases with age and comorbidities. As men with localized disease often do not experience significant disease-related morbidity for many years after diagnosis, and curative treatment itself may result in some morbidity, those with lower-risk cancers and a shorter life expectancy are likely to benefit least from radical treatment.

Active surveillance is becoming increasingly popular, especially for men with small-volume and low-to-moderate-grade prostate cancer (very-low- or low-risk category), who have a low risk of death from

TABLE 5.1

Treatment options for localized and locally advanced cancer

	Localized			
	Risk of recurrence			
Treatment	Low	Intermediate	High	Locally advanced
Radical prostatectomy	✓	✓	✓	Multimodality therapy
EBRT	✓	✓		
EBRT with androgen deprivation		✓	✓	✓
Low-dose seed brachytherapy	✓	✓		
HDR brachytherapy (in combination with EBRT)			✓	✓
Active surveillance	✓			
Watchful waiting	✓	✓	✓	✓
Hormonal therapy			✓	✓
Approaches under investigation				
HIFU	✓			
Cryotherapy	✓			

EBRT, external-beam radiotherapy; HDR, high-dose-rate; HIFU, high-intensity focused ultrasound.

prostate cancer (Table 5.3). These men would be eligible for curative therapy, but this option is deferred until objective signs of disease progression are observed. This approach means the majority of men (60–70%) are spared the side effects of curative therapy when they do not require it.

TABLE 5.2

Categories of risk of recurrence

Risk category	Definition				
	TNM	Gleason score	PSA (ng/mL)	Positive biopsy cores/cancer in each core	PSA density (ng/mL/g)
Very low	T1c	≤ 6	< 10	< 3/< 50%	< 0.15
Low	T1–T2	2–≤ 6	< 10		
Intermediate	T2b–T2c, *or*	7, *or*	10–20		
High	T3a, *or*	8–10, *or*	> 20		

National Comprehensive Cancer Network (NCCN) (guidelines version 3.2013). PSA, prostate-specific antigen; TNM, tumor–nodes–metastasis.

TABLE 5.3

Active surveillance criteria

Active surveillance criteria
Consider men with:
• PSA < 15 ng/mL
• Gleason biopsy score ≤ 3 + 4
• Low volume < 4 mm of any core, and ≤ 3/12 cores involved
• Life expectancy > 10 years/suitable for radical treatment of progression
Confirming:
• 3-Tesla multiparametric MRI showing no index or significant lesion
• Repeat TRUS or transperineal biopsy (if available) within first 6–12 months shows no upgrading or increased volume of cancer
Radical treatment indicated by:
• PSA velocity > 1 ng/mL/year
• Clinical progression on DRE
• Increase in Gleason score on repeat biopsy
• Patient choice

During active surveillance, men are followed closely with regular prostate-specific antigen (PSA) measurement and digital rectal examination (DRE) every 3–6 months. MRI and repeat biopsies are usually organized 6–12 months after diagnosis and when cancer growth is suspected. Increasingly, multiparametric MRI is also being used to select patients for entry or follow-up in active surveillance protocols. Curative therapy is initiated if the cancer shows signs of growth and before the cancer becomes incurable. The cancer-specific survival in men who fit the criteria for active surveillance is 99% at 8 years' follow-up. While men avoid the physical side effects of treatment, they do have to live with the psychological effects of having an untreated cancer, though these do not seem to be troublesome for most men. In most untreated series, only around one-third of men managed by active surveillance progress to active treatment, and those who do are usually cured.

Radical prostatectomy involves surgically removing the entire prostate, the seminal vesicles and a variable amount of adjacent tissue (Figure 5.1). It is appropriate for men for whom it is believed the tumor can be removed completely by surgery, and who satisfy the criteria in Table 5.4. The procedure used to be commonly performed via the retropubic route, but it is now increasingly performed by laparoscopy with robotic assistance. It is possible to also use a perineal approach, but this is falling out of favor. The major advantage of radical prostatectomy is that it excises all prostatic tissue and provides precise histological information and definitive cure in patients in whom the tumor is specimen-confined. Thus, the patient's anxiety is relieved. Given that prostate cancer has a long natural history, this is an important consideration in terms of the patient's quality of life. Long-term studies have shown normal life expectancies in those with complete excision of specimen-confined disease. Ten-year survival for

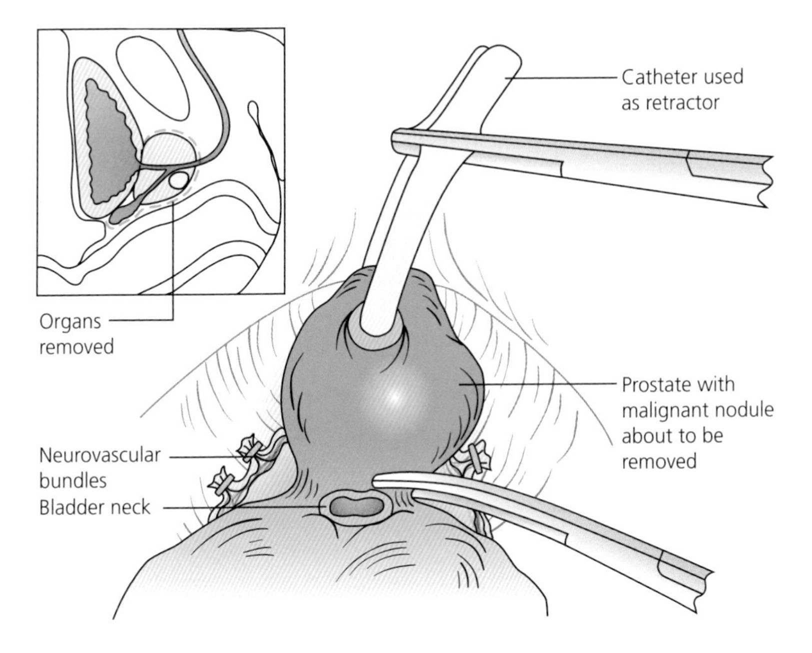

Figure 5.1 Radical prostatectomy. The entire prostate and attached seminal vesicles can be removed surgically and an anastomosis created between the bladder neck and the urethra.

TABLE 5.4

Selection criteria for radical prostatectomy

- Histological evidence of prostate cancer
- Clinically localized disease (stages T1–T2)
- Life expectancy > 10 years
- No contraindications to surgery
- No significant comorbidity

men with clinically localized disease treated with radical prostatectomy is 98%, 91% and 76% for Gleason scores 2–4, 5–7 and 8–10, respectively. Moreover, the procedure also offers definitive treatment of concomitant benign prostatic hyperplasia (BPH) and reliably results in an undetectable PSA.

The principal adverse events associated with radical prostatectomy are stress urinary incontinence (< 2–3%) and erectile dysfunction (> 50%); the latter is age-related, tends to improve with time and can be minimized by nerve-sparing approaches. Moreover, erectile dysfunction after surgery can now be treated quite effectively (see Chapter 9). Table 5.5 summarizes the advantages and disadvantages of radical prostatectomy.

Radical prostatectomy, by whichever means achieved, is believed by most urologists to offer the best opportunity for complete cure in patients with localized prostate cancer. A randomized study from Sweden showed that at a median 8.2 years' follow-up, radical prostatectomy decreased prostate-cancer-related mortality by 44% and overall death by 26% when compared with watchful waiting. The difference was largest in men under 65 years of age. Because the total number of prostate-cancer-related deaths was low, it would require 20 men to undergo prostatectomy to save one man from death.

A similar US study, the Prostate Cancer Intervention Versus Observation Trial (PIVOT), which had a high proportion of low-risk prostate cancers, has reported no observed difference in overall survival with a median follow-up of 10 years, but a 60% reduction in

TABLE 5.5

Advantages and disadvantages of treatment options for localized prostate cancer

Radical prostatectomy

Advantages

- High likelihood of cure if tumor pathologically confined
- Definitive staging possible
- Treatment of concomitant BPH
- Reliable PSA suppression to unrecordable levels
- Side effects improve with time
- Easy monitoring for recurrent disease
- Radiotherapy possible after surgery

Disadvantages

- Major operation
- Potential mortality (< 0.4%)
- Potential morbidity:
  - erectile dysfunction (> 50%)
  - persistent incontinence (< 3%)
  - pulmonary embolism (< 1%)
  - bladder neck stricture (< 5%)
  - infertility

Radiotherapy

Advantages

- Potential cure
- Surgery avoided
- Outpatient therapy

Disadvantages

- Prostate left in situ
- Difficulty assessing cure
- No definitive staging possible
- No benefit for concomitant BPH
- Patient anxiety during follow-up
- Unreliable PSA suppression
- May need androgen deprivation in combination
- Potential morbidity:
  - rectal injury (2–10%)
  - urinary incontinence (< 3%)
  - impotence (20–30%)
  - bladder damage (10–20%)
  - hematuria (5–10%)
- Surgery generally not feasible after radiotherapy

(CONTINUED)

TABLE 5.5 (CONTINUED)

Brachytherapy

Advantages	*Disadvantages*
• One-off treatment • Day-case or overnight procedure • Limited period of catheterization • Low risk of incontinence • Lower risk of erectile dysfunction	• Only appropriate for low-risk disease • Cannot be used after previous prostate surgery • Limited experience of long-term effects • Difficulty assessing cure • Makes subsequent surgery dangerous • Very significant urinary symptoms in first 6 months

prostate cancer mortality for men with high-risk cancers treated with radical prostatectomy. However, the trial has been criticized for under-recruitment and inclusion of very many men with significant comorbidities, leading to an excessive death rate from non-prostate-related causes.

Surgery can also be an effective treatment for high-risk prostate cancer, particularly if it appears to be clinically localized to the prostate gland. In cases of T3 prostate cancer, surgery is appropriate if the cancer can be fully excised. A multimodal approach that includes adjuvant radiotherapy should be considered. Following surgery, patients who have adverse pathological features such as extracapsular extension, seminal vesicle extension or positive margins can be treated with adjuvant radiotherapy to the prostatic bed, often with concomitant androgen ablation. This has been shown, in three randomized trials, to decrease the risk of PSA recurrence by 52% compared with no treatment, and to improve survival. Whether early salvage radiation is equivalent to adjuvant radiation is yet to be answered, and salvage radiotherapy remains an option in these patients (see Chapter 6).

Men having radical prostatectomy for high-risk cancer should also be considered for extended lymph node dissection. This strategy more accurately stages the patient, allowing for better prognostication and institution of adjuvant therapies, and has also been shown to decrease the cancer recurrence and progression rates, as well as possibly improving survival.

Neoadjuvant hormonal therapy prior to radical prostatectomy. Studies have demonstrated reduced PSA levels, prostate volume and tumor volume and also decreased positive surgical margins. However, no advantage in terms of cancer recurrence or survival has been demonstrated and so this practice currently remains investigational.

Robotic-assisted radical prostatectomy (RARP) is increasingly employed (Figure 5.2). Recent systematic reviews and meta-analysis have suggested that oncological outcomes are similar between RARP and open radical prostatectomy. However, urinary incontinence and erectile function recovery at 12 months are perhaps marginally better with RARP. The operating time is usually somewhat longer, but blood

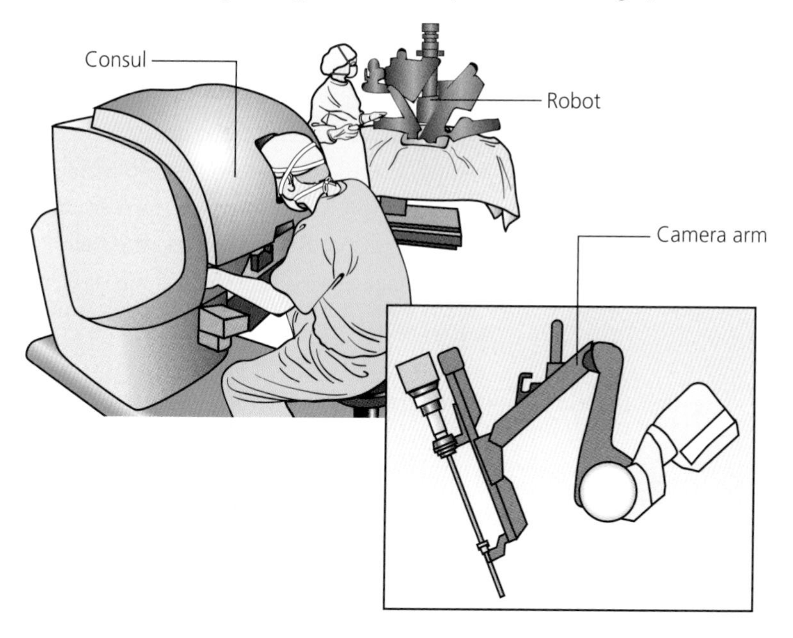

Figure 5.2 Robotic-assisted radical prostatectomy using the da Vinci surgical system.

loss and length of hospital stay are significantly reduced and recovery is quicker. The ten times greater magnification and more precise instrumentation may be responsible for these differences and it certainly makes the surgery very much easier to perform. Patients also return to work more rapidly.

Radiotherapy

External-beam radiotherapy is widely used in the treatment of localized and locally advanced prostate cancer; it offers a particular advantage in patients who are unsuitable for surgery because of comorbidity or evidence of extraprostatic extension of the cancer. Criteria for patients suitable for radiotherapy are shown in Table 5.6. The treatment generally involves a 7.5-week course of three-dimensional conformal radiotherapy or intensity-modulated radiotherapy (IMRT).

The principal side effects are due to changes in the bladder, urethra and rectum that occur as a result of the treatment. In the short term, radiotherapy to the prostate causes frequency of, and stinging on, urination; diarrhea; proctitis; and tiredness. In the longer term, there is a risk of urinary frequency and bleeding, which may occur in severe form in 2–3% of patients. Rectal side effects consist of urgency, frequency, tenesmus and bleeding. Erectile dysfunction due to damage to the neurovascular supply to the corpora cavernosa can also occur, often gradually over a 6–18-month period. Recent advances in the delivery of radiotherapy include image-guided radiotherapy (IGRT),

TABLE 5.6

Selection criteria for external-beam radiotherapy

- Histological evidence of prostate cancer
- Regionally localized disease
- Sufficient life expectancy to make cure potentially beneficial
- Absence of lower urinary tract disorders (particularly outflow obstruction)
- Absence of colorectal disease

whereby gold seed 'fiducial' markers are placed within the prostate so they can be used on a daily basis to focus the radiotherapy beams, increasing radiation delivery to the target and reducing damage to surrounding structures.

A number of studies have shown better cancer control for men with intermediate- or high-risk prostate cancer if the radiation dose is escalated to 74 Gy or higher. The advent of IMRT allows very precise targeting of the prostate, with less radiation scatter to surrounding organs. As a consequence, higher doses can be given to men without a significant increase in local toxicity. The advantages and disadvantages of radiotherapy are summarized in Table 5.5 and are compared with those of radical prostatectomy and brachytherapy.

External-beam radiation alone, that is, without the prior use of hormonal down-sizing therapy, is no longer recommended particularly for patients with intermediate- or high-risk disease. Reduction of the tumor burden with a luteinizing hormone-releasing hormone (LHRH) analog or an antiandrogen appears to increase the sensitivity of cancer cells to death by irradiation. This approach has been validated in randomized trials, where both progression-free and overall survival have been shown to significantly improve when men with high-risk prostate cancers are treated with a combination of external-beam radiotherapy and adjuvant hormonal therapy. In one US trial, the addition of adjuvant hormonal therapy improved overall survival at 10 years from 39.8% to 58.1%. The 10-year prostate cancer mortality was reduced from 30.4% to 10.3% in favor of treatment with radiotherapy and concomitant androgen deprivation therapy (Figure 5.3). Similar improvements have been noted in other North American trials. It is now standard practice to add hormonal therapy to the treatment of all men undergoing external-beam radiotherapy for high-risk disease.

CyberKnife stereotactic body radiation therapy (SBRT) uses computer-assisted image guidance to target around 1200 beams of high-energy radiation to the tumor (Figure 5.4). It can correct for prostate movement, which helps to reduce irradiation of surrounding tissue. Evidence is building to support its use in men with early localized prostate cancer, while there are also early data suggesting it has a role in men with intermediate-risk cancer.

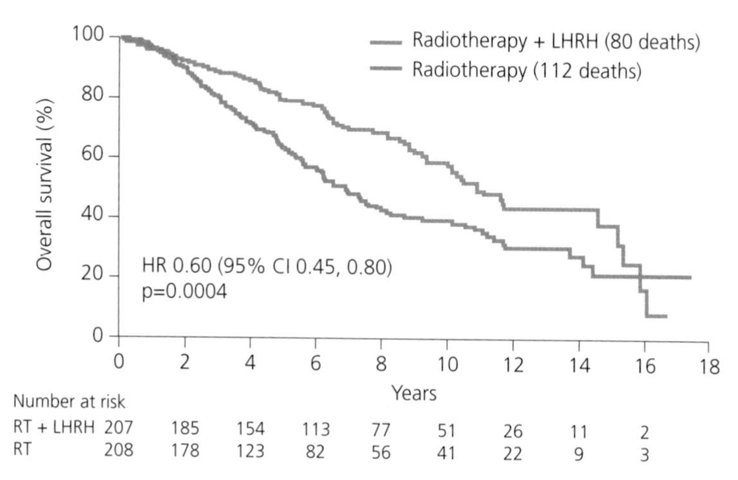

Figure 5.3 In a randomized clinical trial involving men at high metastatic risk, the addition of luteinizing hormone-releasing hormone (LHRH) agonist during and for 3 years after external-beam radiotherapy improved overall survival at 10 years' follow-up. CI, confidence interval; HR, hazard ratio; RT, radiotherapy. Reproduced from Bolla et al., 2010, with permission from Elsevier.

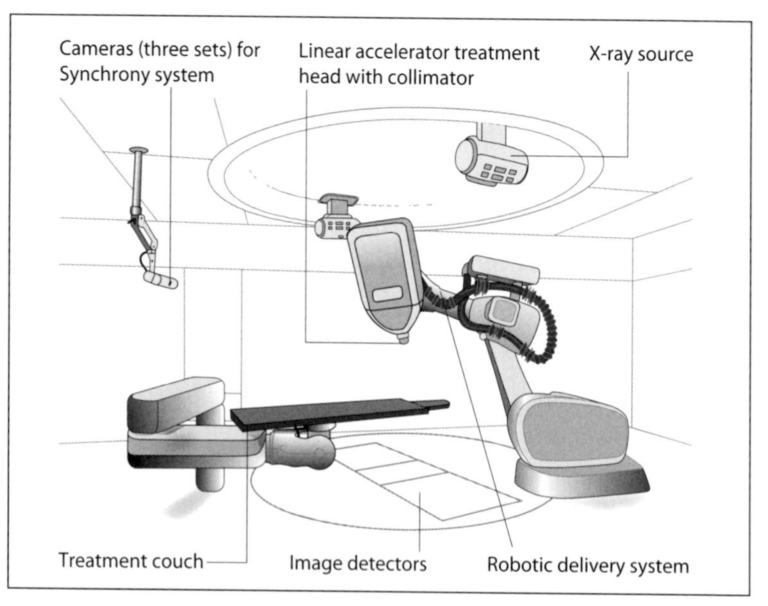

Figure 5.4 The CyberKnife treatment delivery system. Powerful imaging aids accurate targeting of high-energy radiation to the tumor.

Patients tend to appreciate that treatment duration is short, usually only a week. However, longer-term follow-up data are required before CyberKnife becomes an established treatment.

Low-dose seed brachytherapy involves placing either iodine-125 or palladium-103 seeds into the prostate via the transperineal route, using a grid template and transrectal ultrasonography (TRUS) guidance (Figure 5.5). Patient selection criteria are given in Table 5.7.

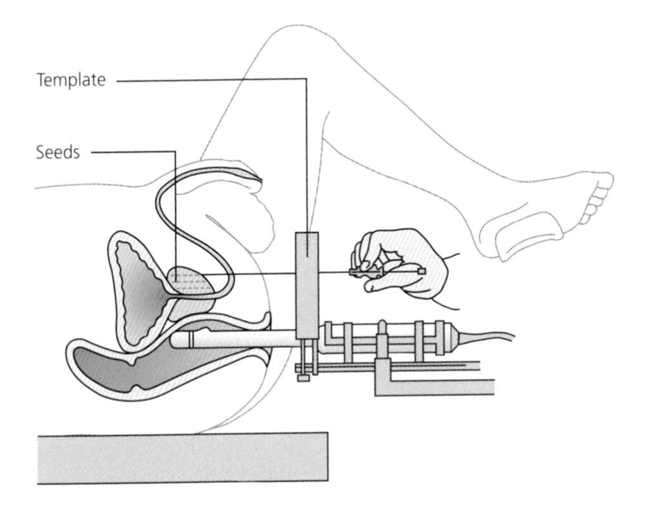

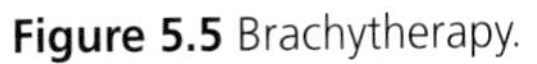
Figure 5.5 Brachytherapy.

TABLE 5.7

Selection criteria for low-dose seed brachytherapy

- Histological evidence of prostate cancer
- Clinically localized disease (T1 or T2)
- Low PSA (preferably < 10 ng/mL)
- Low–moderate Gleason score (2–6) preferable
- Prostate volume not large (< 50 cm^3)
- Minimal obstructive urinary symptoms
- No prior transurethral resection of the prostate (TURP)

The results of seed brachytherapy in low-risk men (PSA < 10 ng/mL, Gleason score < 7 and ≤ cT2b) is equivalent to radical prostatectomy at 10 years, but they are highly dependent on the quality of seed placement. The results in patients with intermediate risk are worse, however, with approximately 66% of men free from recurrence at 10 years.

The method is popular, particularly in the USA, because of its low morbidity; the side effects are similar in nature to those of external-beam radiotherapy, but may also include difficulty with urination because of prostate swelling. In general, brachytherapy is not suitable for prostates with volumes much greater than 50 cm^3 or in men with severe pre-existing bladder outflow obstruction, because these circumstances make seed placement difficult. Previous transurethral resection of the prostate (TURP) is also usually a contraindication to brachytherapy as it is difficult to place the seeds accurately.

High-dose-rate brachytherapy is a relatively new treatment in which a high-intensity iridium source is delivered to the prostate by hollow needles inserted through the perineum (Figure 5.6). It has a number of advantages over low-dose seed brachytherapy.

- The treatment time is very short.
- Very high doses can be achieved in the prostate in a conformal manner (> 96 Gy).
- Dosimetry is determined after insertion of the needles so dosing is much more uniform.
- Treatment with high-dose iridium radiation kills fast-growing tumors more effectively.

High-dose-rate (HDR) brachytherapy can be given as monotherapy or as a prostatic boost in combination with external-beam radiotherapy. The results with the latter combination for intermediate- and high-risk cancer are quite good. The 10-year disease-free survival rate is approximately 69% and cancer-specific survival is 93%. HDR brachytherapy as monotherapy can be used as an alternative to seed brachytherapy. Although only early results are available, cancer control appears to be equivalent, with possibly fewer side effects with HDR brachytherapy.

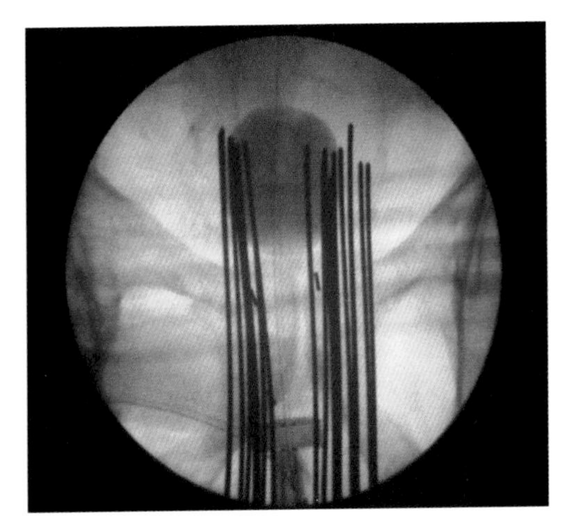

Figure 5.6 An X-ray of a man being treated with high-dose-rate brachytherapy. Needles have been placed in the prostate and the balloon in the catheter has been filled with contrast.

Quality-of-life studies performed on men who have undergone surgery, external-beam radiotherapy or seed brachytherapy show few differences in global quality of life between the different modalities.

Watchful waiting is different from active surveillance in that it is for men who are older or have shorter life expectancy, and who have prostate cancer that is unlikely to shorten their life. These men are counseled and reviewed regularly with clinical examination and PSA measurements. When disease progression is identified, instead of having curative therapy, palliative androgen deprivation is initiated. This is continued until death. In a recent meta-analysis, the development of metastatic disease during watchful waiting was reported to be 2.1% per year in patients with well-differentiated tumors (Gleason scores 2–4), compared with 13.5% per year in patients with aggressive tumors (Gleason scores 7–10). In another study, patients with low-grade tumors treated with watchful waiting had a 92% disease-specific survival at 10 years compared with 76% and 43% for moderate-grade and high-grade tumors, respectively.

Men with high-risk prostate cancer are at higher risk of prostate cancer-specific mortality. However, if significant comorbidities are present, watchful waiting may still be the most appropriate treatment option as they will not infrequently succumb to other comorbid conditions. Patients and their immediate family should be fully informed about the implications of opting for watchful waiting; PSA values should be monitored carefully and symptomatic treatment offered as appropriate in these men.

High-intensity focused ultrasound (HIFU) technology has been developed to treat localized prostate cancer. A probe delivers HIFU transrectally to the prostate and achieves focal tissue destruction (Figure 5.7). Early results are promising, with around three-quarters of men with low-risk disease reported to be disease free at 5 years' follow-up in some series. HIFU can also be used for the treatment of cancer recurrence after radiotherapy. The method should currently be regarded as experimental, particularly as side effects of incontinence and the development of urinary fistula may be troublesome and are often difficult to resolve. The reliability and durability of this treatment is still uncertain.

Cryoablation. Freezing temperatures can be used to destroy prostatic tissue. Under TRUS guidance, a number of cryogenic probes are inserted into the prostate via the perineum (Figure 5.8). Liquid nitrogen is then circulated through the probes, producing 'ice balls' with a temperature of approximately –180°C that disrupt cell membranes, thereby destroying the surrounding tissue. The urethra is protected by circulating warm (44°C) water through a catheter. Although some studies have reported outcomes comparable to those

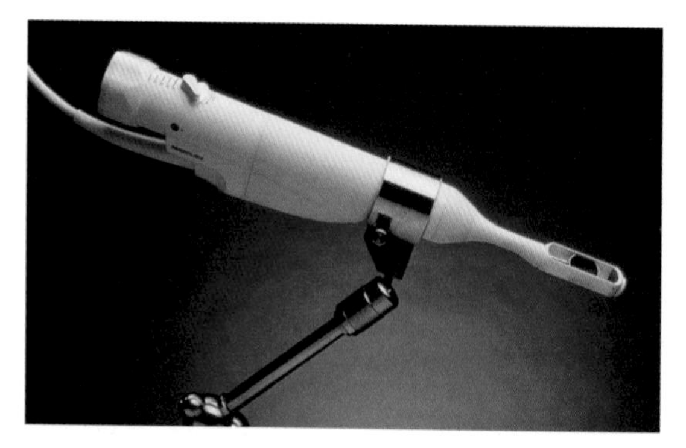

Figure 5.7 High-intensity focused ultrasound (HIFU) probe for endorectal treatment of localized prostate cancer.

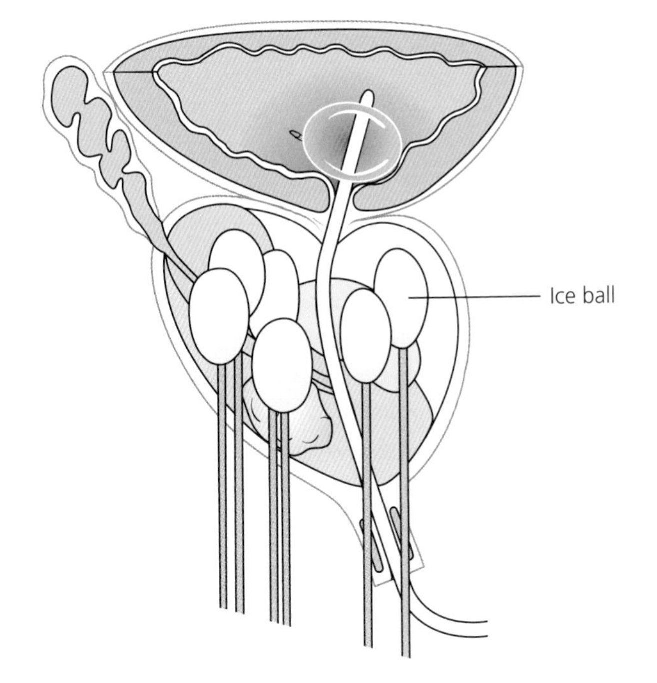

Figure 5.8 In cryoablation, cryogenic probes are inserted into the prostate under ultrasound guidance. Liquid nitrogen is circulated through the probes, forming 'ice balls', which destroy prostatic tissue. The urethra is protected by warming through a catheter.

achieved by radical prostatectomy, others have reported a significant incidence of complications such as rectal and urethral damage. No long-term randomized controlled trials have yet compared cryoablation with more established treatments, and the treatment may be more applicable to patients with recurrence after radiotherapy, though prostate–rectal fistulae remain a problem.

Hormonal treatment alone. A full discussion of hormonal therapy is given in Chapter 7. Conventional hormone ablation therapy for locally advanced prostate cancer (T3 or T4 prostate cancer) involves the use of depot LHRH analogs, preceded and accompanied by an antiandrogen for at least 2–6 weeks and sometimes continued thereafter for a period of up to 3 years.

Monotherapy with antiandrogens. Monotherapy with the antiandrogen bicalutamide, 150 mg/day, has been shown in randomized trials to be as effective in controlling locally advanced disease as castration treatment by either orchidectomy or LHRH analog. In addition, in a very large international randomized trial, with median follow-up of 7.4 years, adjuvant treatment with bicalutamide, 150 mg/day, plus standard therapy for locally advanced prostate cancer (i.e. surgery, radiotherapy or watchful waiting) significantly reduced objective progression by 31% when compared with placebo plus standard therapy. A survival benefit of 35% was also observed in men undergoing radiation with adjuvant bicalutamide. The advantage of using the antiandrogen option is that sexual interest and function may be preserved (Figure 5.9). Younger patients may often opt for treatment that has a lesser impact on this important aspect of their lives. They should be warned, however, that gynecomastia is likely. If progression occurs, treatment with an LHRH analog may give beneficial results.

Management of local complications. Locally advanced prostate cancer may cause any of several urologic emergencies. Acute or chronic urinary retention may require TURP. Care should be taken with this

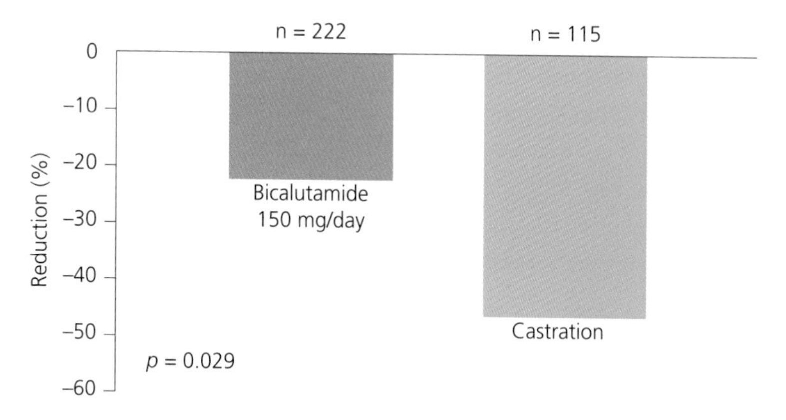

Figure 5.9 Percentage reduction from baseline in sexual interest after 12 months' treatment: bicalutamide, 150 mg/day, versus castration in M0 patients. Adapted from Iversen P. *Eur Urol* 1999;36(suppl 2):20–6.

procedure not to induce urinary incontinence because the normal landmarks can be distorted by the tumor. A period of catheter drainage during androgen ablation, followed by a trial without the catheter, is often indicated before surgery.

Anuria resulting from bilateral ureteric obstruction, either at the vesico–ureteric junction or at the pelvic brim due to enlarged lymph nodes, may necessitate insertion of nephrostomy tubes or passage of a double-pigtail stent and subsequent external-beam radiotherapy.

Bleeding from the tumor may occasionally precipitate hematuria and clot retention, requiring bladder washout and irrigation, and sometimes diathermy or even embolization of bleeding tumor vessels.

Key points – management of localized and high-risk disease

- The treatment of localized prostate cancer is controversial.
- Active surveillance is increasingly used for very-low- and low-risk disease.
- Approximately one-third of men managed with active surveillance go on to receive curative treatment.
- Radical prostatectomy probably offers the best prospect of long-term cure, but carries the disadvantage of possible sexual dysfunction and incontinence.
- In the case of high-risk cancer, surgery may be considered as one part of a multimodal therapeutic approach.
- External-beam radiotherapy can be curative, but is associated with possible rectal and bladder complications.
- Brachytherapy can be combined with external-beam radiotherapy in higher-risk individuals.
- Treatment with external-beam radiotherapy and hormonal therapy is more effective than radiotherapy alone.
- Local staging by MRI may be helpful in men with intermediate- or high-risk prostate cancer.
- In a large international trial, ongoing treatment with the antiandrogen bicalutamide, 150 mg/day, reduced objective progression by 31%, but gynecomastia was common.

Key references

Albertsen PC, Hanley JA, Fine J. 20-year outcomes following conservative management of clinically localized prostate cancer. *JAMA* 2005;293:2095–101.

Bill-Axelson A, Holmberg L, Ruutu M et al. Radical prostatectomy versus watchful waiting in early prostate cancer. *N Engl J Med* 2005;352:1977–84.

Bolla M, Van Tienhoven G, Warde P et al. External irradiation with or without long-term androgen suppression for prostate cancer with high metastatic risk: 10-year results of an EORTC randomised study. *Lancet Oncol* 2010;11:1066–73.

D'Amico AV, Chen MH, Renshaw AA et al. Androgen suppression and radiation vs radiation alone for prostate cancer: a randomized trial. *JAMA* 2008;299:289–95.

D'Amico AV, Denham JW, Bolla M et al. Short- vs long-term androgen suppression plus external beam radiation therapy and survival in men of advanced age with node-negative high-risk adenocarcinoma of the prostate. *Cancer* 2007;109:2004–10.

Holmberg L, Bill-Axelson A, Helgesen F et al. A randomized trial comparing radical prostatectomy with watchful waiting in early prostate cancer. *N Engl J Med* 2002;347:781–9.

Klotz L, Zhang L, Lam A et al. Clinical results of long-term follow-up of a large, active surveillance cohort with localized prostate cancer. *J Clin Oncol* 2010;28:126–31.

Stephenson AJ, Scardino PT, Kattan MW et al. Predicting the outcome of salvage radiation therapy for recurrent prostate cancer after radical prostatectomy. *J Clin Oncol* 2007;25:2035–41.

Thompson IM, Tangen CM, Paradelo J et al. Adjuvant radiotherapy for pathological T3N0M0 prostate cancer significantly reduces risk of metastases and improves survival: long-term followup of a randomized clinical trial. *J Urol* 2009;181:956–62.

Uchida T, Ohkusa H, Yamashita H et al. Five years experience of transrectal high-intensity focused ultrasound using the Sonablate device in the treatment of localized prostate cancer. *Int J Urol* 2006;13:228–33.

Wilt TJ, Brawer MK, Jones KM et al. Radical prostatectomy versus observation for localized prostate cancer. *N Engl J Med* 2012;367:203–13.

6 Managing recurrence after initial therapy

Following initial treatment – surgery or radiotherapy – recurrence usually manifests itself as a rise in the prostate-specific antigen (PSA). Digital rectal examination, CT scan or MRI and bone scan are the next steps, but unless the PSA level is significantly raised, these tests may not reveal a specific site. The ProstaScint scan, which is based on a radioimmunoassay for prostate-specific membrane antigen, may reveal sites of metastases not identified by other means but sometimes gives false-positive results; the investigation is still regarded as experimental. A choline positron emission tomography (PET)/CT scan may be more informative (see page 51).

Recurrence following prostatectomy

Of men undergoing radical prostatectomy, 15–46% suffer eventual cancer recurrence in the form of a postoperative rise in PSA. Risk factors for recurrence include:

- positive surgical margins
- extracapsular extension
- seminal vesicle involvement, and/or
- lymph node metastases at the time of surgery.

Following prostatectomy, the PSA level should reliably fall to below 0.1 ng/mL. The recommendations for cut-off values to indicate cancer recurrence range from 0.2 ng/mL to 0.5 ng/mL. If the PSA level does not fall to below this level within 6 weeks postoperatively, the presence of systemic disease should be considered.

Cancer recurrence is confirmed once a patient has a PSA level that is above the cut-off and rising, but time to metastasis and death is variable and often quite prolonged. On average, a patient with a PSA recurrence will develop metastases over a median of 8 years, with death 5 years after the development of metastases. A number of factors determine how fast the cancer recurrence will actually progress:

- time to recurrence after prostatectomy, as a shorter time to recurrence is associated with faster progression of disease

- time it takes for the PSA to double, as a doubling time of less than 3 months is associated with shorter time to metastases and death
- Gleason score.

When cancer recurs by PSA level only, it is not known whether the recurrence is local (in the prostate bed) or systemic (metastases). A number of factors can also help with estimation of the likelihood of local versus systemic disease (Table 6.1).

The management of PSA recurrence consists of a number of choices. These include watchful waiting, salvage radiotherapy and hormonal therapy.

Watchful waiting is ideal for the man with a limited life expectancy and/or lower probability of disease progression based on the earlier criteria. It should be remembered that, in the average patient, metastases do not develop until 8 years after a PSA rise is detected, with death 5 years later.

Salvage radiotherapy is a potentially curative treatment option for men with a high likelihood of residual cancer in the prostatic bed. The best results are in those men who have a Gleason score of 7 or lower, pre-radiotherapy PSA below 1.0 ng/mL, positive surgical margins and a PSA doubling time of more than 10 months. The effectiveness of salvage radiation is improving, with 60–90% of men achieving

TABLE 6.1

PSA and pathology variables that predict local or systemic recurrence following radical prostatectomy

Variable	Local recurrence	Systemic recurrence
Gleason score	≤ 7	> 7
Lymph node invasion	No	Yes
PSA doubling time	> 12 months	< 3 months
Seminal vesicle involvement	No	Yes
Time to PSA recurrence	> 1 year	< 1 year

undetectable PSA levels, especially if concomitant androgen ablation is employed.

Side effects include possible loss of erectile function, bladder neck contracture and proctitis. Androgen ablation with an antiandrogen or luteinizing hormone-releasing hormone (LHRH) analog is increasingly used to enhance the effectiveness of the radiation treatment and can continue for 12–24 months.

Hormonal therapy is reserved for men who have progressive PSA rises and are unlikely to harbor isolated local recurrence. In these men, who have presumed systemic disease, the timing of the commencement of hormonal therapy is controversial. There is evidence that hormonal therapy started early in patients with an asymptomatic increase in PSA results has delayed development of bone metastases, but it has not been unequivocally shown to improve survival. For more information on hormone therapy, see Chapter 7.

Recurrence following radiation therapy

The definition of recurrence after radiation treatment is less straightforward than that after surgery. Following radiation, the PSA falls slowly over 12–24 months to a nadir at detectable levels, usually below 1.0 ng/mL. In addition, approximately 30% of men have a transient rise (a 'bounce'). To complicate matters further, adjuvant hormonal therapy is often used, which suppresses PSA, but once it is stopped the PSA slowly rises as the testosterone levels rise.

Currently, recurrence after radiation therapy is defined as PSA 2 ng/mL above the nadir level. The natural history of PSA recurrence is not as clear in patients who have had radiation therapy as in those who have had surgery. PSA doubling time is clearly the best predictor of metastatic disease, and in fact a PSA doubling time of less than 3 months is also associated with a higher risk of death.

Once a PSA recurrence has been defined, further investigations depend on the individual's circumstances and expectations and involve determining whether the cancer is present in the prostate or is systemic, or both. ProstaScint imaging can be used in addition to the staging imaging of a bone scan and CT or MRI, though it is still considered experimental. A choline PET/CT scan may reveal the location of the recurrence. A prostate re-biopsy can be performed if salvage treatment for local disease is being considered, but the result is often negative.

There are several options for treatment. Watchful waiting can be offered to men who have limited life expectancy and/or slow progression of their cancer. Salvage prostatectomy is an option for men who are likely to have cancer limited to the prostate, but it is considerably more difficult than in men who have not had radiation and has a significantly higher incidence of side effects. Cryotherapy and high-intensity focused ultrasound (HIFU) therapy are also options

Key points – managing recurrence after initial therapy

- PSA level should reliably fall to below 0.1 ng/mL following prostatectomy.
- Recurrence after prostatectomy is generally defined as PSA above 0.2 ng/mL and rising.
- Recurrence after radiation therapy is usually defined as PSA 2 ng/mL above the nadir level.
- For the average patient, metastases do not develop until 8 years after a PSA rise is detected, so watchful waiting is an appropriate option for some men with recurrence.
- Following prostatectomy, patients who have a high likelihood of local disease can be offered salvage radiotherapy.
- Following radiotherapy, patients who have recurrence in the prostate only may be offered a salvage treatment such as radical prostatectomy, high-intensity focused ultrasound (HIFU) or cryotherapy, but all of these carry the risk of side effects.
- Progressive PSA rises following initial therapy, which suggest the presence of micro-metastatic disease, should be treated with hormone therapy; however, the timing of this treatment is controversial.
- More evidence is needed from clinical trials to inform us of the best treatment options.

but carry significant risks of complications. Hormonal therapy is usually reserved for men who are unlikely to have isolated localized disease. As with hormone therapy after prostatectomy, the timing of hormone therapy for recurrence after radiation therapy is still controversial.

Key references

Bianco FJ Jr, Scardino PT, Stephenson AJ et al. Long-term oncologic results of salvage radical prostatectomy for locally recurrent prostate cancer after radiotherapy. *Int J Radiat Oncol Biol Phys* 2005;62:448–53.

D'Amico AV, Moul J, Carroll PR et al. Prostate specific antigen doubling time as a surrogate end point for prostate cancer specific mortality following radical prostatectomy or radiation therapy. *J Urol* 2004;172:S42–6.

Freedland SJ, Humphreys EB, Mangold LA et al. Risk of prostate cancer-specific mortality following biochemical recurrence after radical prostatectomy. *JAMA* 2005;294:433–9.

Pound CR, Partin AW, Eisenberger MA et al. Natural history of progression after PSA elevation following radical prostatectomy. *JAMA* 1999;281:1591–7.

Roach M 3rd, Hanks G, Thames H Jr et al. Defining biochemical failure following radiotherapy with or without hormonal therapy in men with clinically localized prostate cancer: recommendations of the RTOG-ASTRO Phoenix Consensus Conference. *Int J Radiat Oncol Biol Phys* 2006;65:965–74.

Stephenson AJ, Scardino PT, Kattan MW et al. Predicting the outcome of salvage radiation therapy for recurrent prostate cancer after radical prostatectomy. *J Clin Oncol* 2007;25:2035–41.

Stephenson AJ, Shariat SF, Zelefsky MJ et al. Salvage radiotherapy for recurrent prostate cancer after radical prostatectomy. *JAMA* 2004;291:1325–32.

Thompson IM, Tangen CM, Paradelo J et al. Adjuvant radiotherapy for pathological T3N0M0 prostate cancer significantly reduces risk of metastases and improves survival: long-term followup of a randomized clinical trial. *J Urol* 2009;181: 956–62.

Trock BJ, Han M, Freedland SJ et al. Prostate-specific survival following salvage radiotherapy vs observation in men with biochemical recurrence after radical prostatectomy. *JAMA* 2008;299:2760–9.

Van der Kwast TH, Bolla M, Van Poppel H et al. Identification of patients with prostate cancer who benefit from immediate postoperative radiotherapy: EORTC 22911. *J Clin Oncol* 2007;25: 4178–86.

7 Management of metastatic prostate cancer

Although there is a trend towards earlier detection of prostate cancer, many men throughout the world still present with metastatic disease. In countries where prostate-specific antigen (PSA) testing is not widely used, around 30% of patients present with localized disease, 40% with locally advanced disease and the remaining 30% with metastases. In contrast to localized or locally advanced disease, metastatic prostate cancer is associated with high mortality – approximately 70% within 5 years. Androgen deprivation, which has become the mainstay of treatment, effectively reduces intratumoral dihydrotestosterone (DHT) concentration by 70–80%, resulting in reduced androgen-receptor stimulation and increased prostate cancer apoptosis (Table 7.1). Androgen deprivation can be achieved by orchidectomy or treatment with luteinizing hormone-releasing hormone (LHRH) analogs/ antagonists, and the value of adding an antiandrogen (maximal androgen blockade) is still debated.

Some of the trials with important results for the treatment of metastatic prostate cancer are summarized at the end of this chapter (see Table 7.4).

TABLE 7.1

Treatment options for metastatic prostate cancer

- Androgen deprivation
  - orchidectomy
  - LHRH analogs
  - LHRH antagonists
- Maximal androgen blockade
- Intermittent androgen blockade

LHRH, luteinizing hormone-releasing hormone.

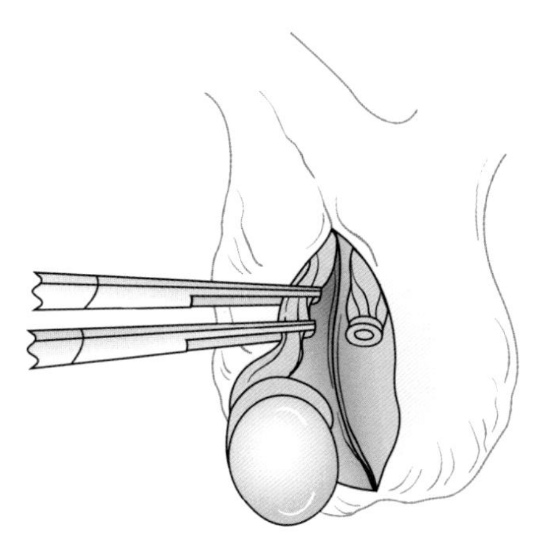

Figure 7.1 Bilateral orchidectomy is generally performed via a midline scrotal incision.

Orchidectomy

Bilateral orchidectomy or bilateral subcapsular orchidectomy is performed through a midline scrotal incision (Figure 7.1) under local, regional or light general anesthesia. The procedure is simple and is associated with little morbidity. The principal adverse events that may occur after orchidectomy are local complications such as hematoma and wound infections, together with general complications of androgen deprivation such as loss of libido, erectile dysfunction and hot flashes (Table 7.2). Clinical responses (decreased bone pain and reduced PSA concentration) are obtained in more than 75% of

TABLE 7.2

Side effects of androgen-deprivation therapy

- Hot flashes
- Decreased libido
- Lethargy
- Cognitive decline
- Mood changes
- Osteoporosis
- Weight gain
- Loss of muscle mass

patients. Because of the psychological/cosmetic impact of orchidectomy and its irreversibility, however, most patients and their partners prefer non-surgical treatment with LHRH analogs/antagonists.

Luteinizing hormone-releasing hormone analogs

LHRH analogs, such as goserelin acetate, buserelin and leuprorelin (leuprolide acetate), are highly potent LHRH agonists (superagonists). After administration, there is a transient initial increase in luteinizing hormone (LH) secretion, and hence in testosterone secretion; this is followed by desensitization (downregulation), resulting in a fall in LH and testosterone secretion (Figure 7.2). These agents can be delivered via 1- , 3- or 6-monthly depot preparations, administered

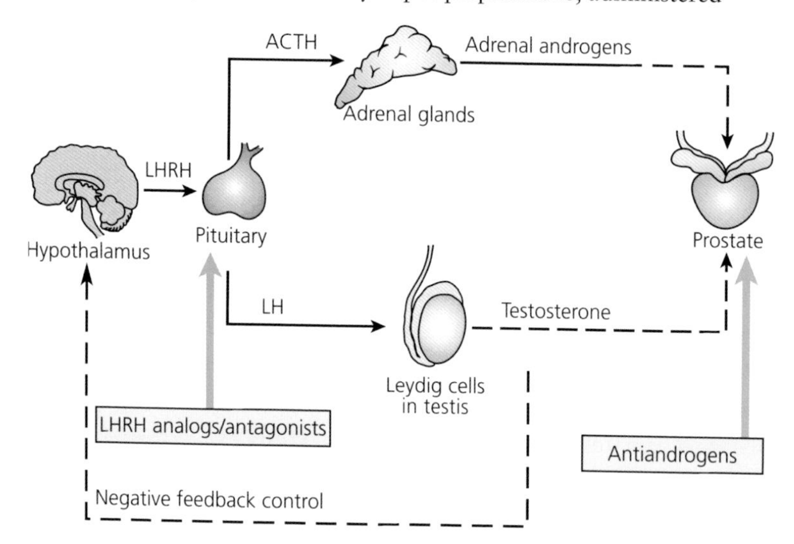

Figure 7.2 Luteinizing hormone-releasing hormone (LHRH) analogs initially stimulate the release of luteinizing hormone (LH) and thus testosterone secretion ('hormone flare') but then desensitize the pituitary LHRH receptors, resulting in a fall in LH, and thus testosterone, levels. LHRH antagonists compete with naturally occurring LHRH to bind to the pituitary LHRH receptors, preventing the release of LH. This leads to a rapid suppression of testosterone release from the testes. Antiandrogens act peripherally to block testosterone action on androgen receptors. ACTH, adrenocorticotropic hormone.

subcutaneously or intramuscularly. A potential side effect is tumor 'flare', which 8–32% of patients experience as a result of the initial transient increase (140–170%) in testosterone. This may result in increased bone pain or worsening of symptoms of bladder outflow or ureteric obstruction; spinal metastases may also be stimulated, increasing a risk of spinal cord compression. Tumor flare can be avoided by prior and concomitant administration of an antiandrogen during the first 4–6 weeks of treatment. Comparative trials have shown that the response rates obtained with LHRH analogs are equivalent to those obtained after orchidectomy in terms of time to progression and overall survival. The reduction of testosterone that results from treatment with these agents may induce features of the metabolic syndrome.

Luteinizing hormone-releasing hormone antagonists

Pure LHRH (or gonadotropin-releasing hormone [GnRH]) antagonists have been developed and evaluated. These peptides inhibit LHRH release without causing the initial stimulation seen with LHRH analogs by blocking pituitary receptors; thus they are not associated with a surge in testosterone (flare). The LHRH antagonist abarelix has shown positive clinical results in controlled clinical studies involving men with hormone-sensitive prostate cancer, as has degarelix (Figure 7.3). A rapid reduction in testosterone without flare was achieved with both antagonists, compared with the significant flare resulting from the administration of an LHRH analog. PSA rapidly decreased in both cases and this effect was maintained in the long term with both agents.

Abarelix has been associated with occasional hypersensitivity; degarelix seldom causes this problem. LHRH antagonists are particularly beneficial for patients with bony metastases, spinal cord compression or bladder neck obstruction, for whom rapid tumor control without testosterone surge is important. An additional potential benefit could be in men receiving intermittent hormonal therapy, in whom the rapid return to LHRH receptor function following withdrawal of the drug results in an accompanying rapid return of testosterone. Recently, it has been suggested that LHRH antagonists carry a lower risk of cardiovascular side effects.

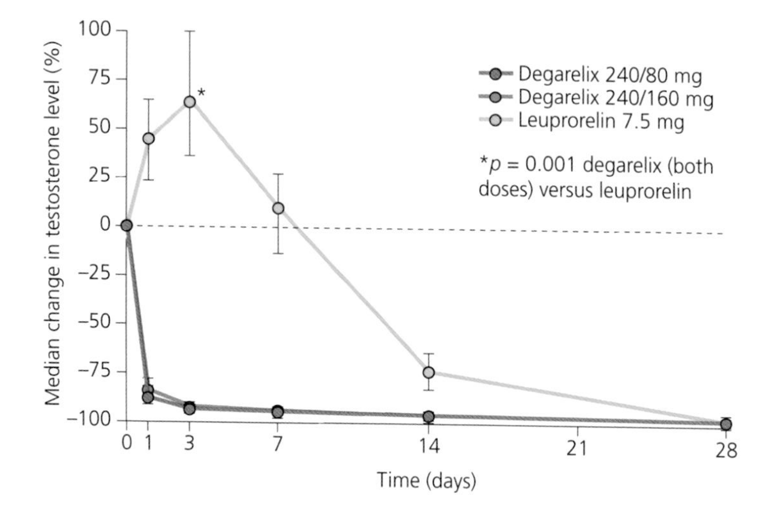

Figure 7.3 The effect of luteinizing hormone-releasing hormone (LHRH) antagonist on testosterone level. Degarelix at a starting dose of 240 mg followed by a monthly maintenance dose of either 80 mg or 160 mg reduced serum testosterone level more rapidly than leuprorelin at the standard monthly dose of 7.5 mg. This phase III trial involved 610 men with prostate cancer (any stage). Reproduced with permission from Klotz et al. 2008.

Antiandrogens

Antiandrogens are taken in tablet form and do not alter the levels of circulating androgens. Instead, they inhibit the androgen receptor where testosterone or DHT binds. There are two classes of these drugs.

- The steroidal antiandrogens (e.g. cyproterone acetate) also have a central testosterone-lowering effect and can be taken as monotherapy instead of castration, although they are not as effective.
- The non-steroidal antiandrogens inhibit the androgen receptor only and should not be taken as monotherapy for metastatic disease as the results are inferior to those achieved with LHRH analogs.

Maximal androgen blockade

Although both orchidectomy and LHRH treatment produce dramatic initial responses in 70–80% of men, remission is not usually maintained in the long term. Androgen-independent cancer cell clones are selected out, so the mean time to tumor progression is less than 18 months and the mean overall survival time is 28–36 months. One factor that may contribute to this poor prognosis is persistent adrenal androgen secretion; there is evidence that adrenal androgens account for up to 15–20% of total androgen concentrations within the prostate. This has led to the concept of 'maximal androgen blockade', in which androgen deprivation by orchidectomy or LHRH treatment is accompanied by treatment with an antiandrogen to block the effects of adrenal androgens in the prostate.

Maximal androgen blockade with a combination of an LHRH analog and an antiandrogen has been shown in several trials to offer improved survival compared with either LHRH analog treatment alone or orchidectomy. However, other trials have failed to show significant improvements in tumor progression and survival, and a meta-analysis of all studies demonstrated little or no advantage for combined therapy. This discrepancy may arise from steroidal and non-steroidal antiandrogens being evaluated together. A subgroup analysis of combination treatment with non-steroidal antiandrogens showed a small survival advantage – 2.9% – for combination therapy compared with monotherapy.

In addition, maximal androgen blockade may offer a slight advantage over monotherapy, at least in a subgroup of patients with good performance status (i.e. those who are generally well in themselves) and a relatively restricted metastatic burden. Such treatment should, therefore, be considered in younger and fitter patients who are most likely to die from prostate cancer itself rather than from some comorbid condition. However, the relatively modest benefits need to be weighed against the increased costs and the small but significant incidence in side effects from the antiandrogens.

The timing of hormonal therapy has been the subject of vigorous debate. The evidence now seems to favor earlier therapy rather than waiting for symptoms. This evidence includes a re-analysis of the cooperative studies (USA) in which men receiving 1 mg of diethylstilbestrol (DES) had a survival advantage. The Medical Research Council (UK) study showed that men with locally advanced or metastatic disease treated with castration at the time of diagnosis had better outcomes than those receiving deferred therapy (Figure 7.4; Table 7.3), and a US trial reported by Messing et al. found that men with pelvic lymph node metastases treated with delayed hormonal therapy had a sevenfold increase in deaths from prostate cancer compared with those who had immediate androgen ablation therapy.

It is clear that early initiation of hormone therapy in men with locally advanced or metastatic disease improves survival and decreases complications. It is not yet clear how early we should start hormone therapy in men who have rising PSA following primary treatment with surgery or radiotherapy in the absence of demonstrable metastases, even though it is expected that the rising PSA is from metastases. It should be borne in mind, however, that earlier treatment with hormonal therapy increases the risk of side effects such as osteoporosis.

Intermittent hormonal therapy

It has been suggested that continuous androgen ablation therapy may, in fact, increase the rate of progression of prostate cancer to a castrate-resistant state (see Chapter 8). For this reason, attention is focused on the use of intermittent hormonal therapy, which also has the potential advantage of decreasing the side effects of therapy. In this approach, hormone therapy is initially given for 6–9 months. Intermittent therapy becomes an option for men in whom there is a response to therapy with PSA levels becoming normalized, and their LHRH analog/antagonist therapy is temporarily discontinued.

Hormone therapy is resumed when the serum PSA concentration returns to pretreatment levels in patients with a PSA at diagnosis below 20 ng/mL, or when PSA increases to more than 20 ng/mL in patients with an initial PSA above this. Such a regimen allows serum testosterone to return to normal, thereby stimulating atrophic cells and rendering them more sensitive to androgen ablation (Figure 7.5). The use of a pure LHRH antagonist, which blocks the receptor

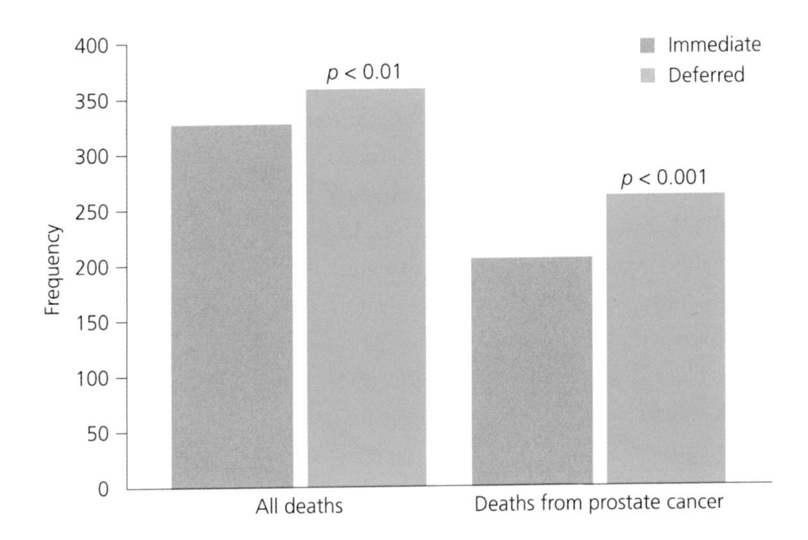

Figure 7.4 Immediate hormonal therapy versus deferred treatment for advanced prostate cancer. Adapted from the Medical Research Council Prostate Cancer Working Party Investigators Group. *Br J Urol* 1997;79: 235–46.

TABLE 7.3

Prostate-cancer-related complications in men with locally advanced or metastatic disease randomized to immediate or delayed hormone therapy*

	Immediate hormone therapy (n = 469)	Delayed hormone therapy (n = 465)
Pathological fracture	11	21
Cord compression	9	23
Ureteric obstruction	33	55
Development of extraskeletal metastases	37	55

*Adapted from the Medical Research Council Prostate Cancer Working Party Investigators Group 1997.

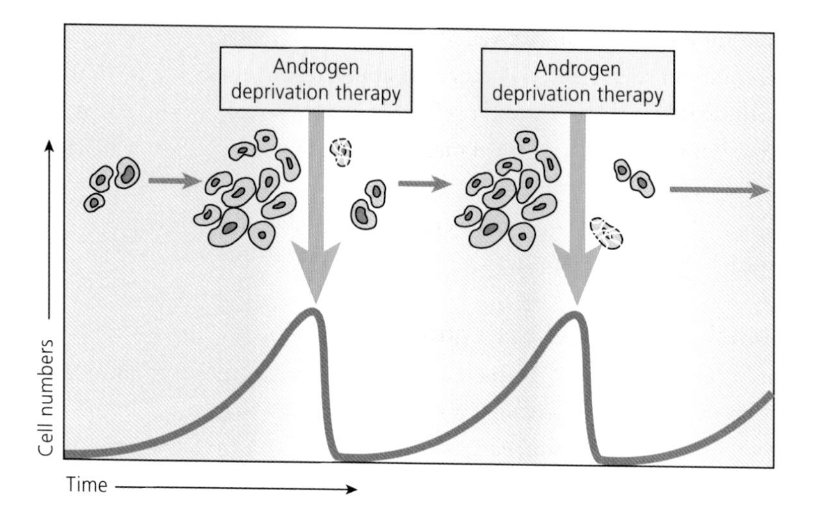

Figure 7.5 Intermittent androgen ablation therapy allows serum testosterone to return periodically to normal, thereby stimulating atrophic cells and rendering them sensitive to subsequent androgen ablation.

without initial stimulation, could be advantageous in this setting owing to the absence of flare and potentially a more rapid restoration of testosterone level after cessation of therapy. In some studies of intermittent hormonal therapy, up to five treatment cycles have been given before evidence of castrate resistance has appeared, and during this time men have spent approximately 50% of the time off therapy.

Two randomized trials of intermittent versus continuous treatment in men with advanced prostate cancer have been published. The first study from Canada, which included 1386 men with a rising PSA after failure of radiotherapy, randomized men to continuous versus intermittent hormone therapy. There was no difference in survival between the two groups, and men survived for approximately 9 years. The group receiving intermittent treatment did, however, show improved quality of life in the areas of physical function, fatigue, hot flashes, libido and erectile function. The results from a US study of 1535 men with metastatic prostate cancer randomized to continuous versus intermittent hormone treatment were statistically inconclusive, although there was a trend for longer survival in men receiving continuous treatment (5.8 years) compared with men receiving intermittent treatment (5.1 years). It appears that intermittent hormone therapy is safe and preferable in men simply with a rising PSA, but men with confirmed metastatic disease may be better treated with continuous therapy.

See Chapter 9 for the management of the adverse effects of androgen-deprivation therapy.

Spinal cord compression and pathological fractures

Sudden onset of low back pain and weakness in the lower limbs, with or without voiding difficulty, in a patient with metastatic prostate cancer should be considered to be a urologic/neurosurgical emergency. Spinal cord compression due to pathological fracture or collapse of the lumbar vertebrae is the most common reason for these symptoms (Figure 7.6). The diagnosis may be confirmed by urgent spinal MRI. Early neurosurgical decompression is often advised, usually followed by external-beam radiotherapy and corticosteroids.

Pathological fractures caused by prostate cancer metastases may occur elsewhere, for example in the femur or humerus. Fixation by an orthopedic specialist is often required and should usually be followed by external-beam radiotherapy and androgen ablation.

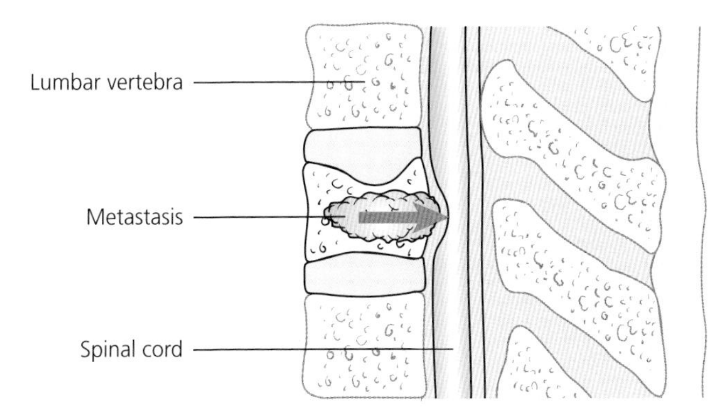

Figure 7.6 Spinal cord compression as a result of a spinal metastasis.

TABLE 7.4

Important trials in the treatment of metastatic prostate cancer

Medication	Comparator	Use	Trial	Key outcomes
LHRH agonist	Orchidectomy	Metastatic prostate cancer	Seidenfeld et al., 2000	• Systematic review and meta-analysis of ten trials • LHRH agonist demonstrated equivalent survival to orchidectomy (HR 1.12 [0.91–1.39])
Maximal androgen blockade (MAB)	Monotherapy androgen suppression	Metastatic prostate cancer	[Prostate Cancer Trialists' Collaborative Group], 2000	• Meta-analysis of 27 trials and 8275 men • 2.9% survival increase for men treated with MAB (non-steroidal) versus monotherapy • 2.8% survival decrease if MAB with cyproterone acetate used
Early hormonal therapy	Delayed hormonal therapy	Locally advanced and metastatic prostate cancer	[The Medical Research Council Prostate Cancer Working Party Investigators Group], 1997	• Randomized trial of 938 men • 257 men died from prostate cancer in the delayed arm versus 203 in the early treatment arm (p=0.001) • The difference was largely seen in the men with stage C disease • Complications from prostate cancer were almost halved in men on the immediate arm

CONTINUED

TABLE 7.4 (CONTINUED)

Medication	Comparator	Use	Trial	Key outcomes
Early hormonal therapy	Delayed hormonal therapy	Men with pathologically involved lymph nodes after radical prostatectomy	Messing et al., 2006	• 98 men randomized to early versus delayed hormone therapy • At 11.9 years' follow-up there was significant improvement in overall survival (HR 1.84 [1.01–3.35]); prostate-cancer-specific survival (HR 4.09 [1.76–9.49])
Intermittent hormone therapy	Continuous hormone therapy	Men with rising PSA after radiotherapy	Crook et al., 2012	• 1386 men randomized to intermittent versus continuous hormone therapy • Intermittent: significant quality of life benefits • Median survival 8.8 years for intermittent versus 9.1 years for continuous (not significant)
Intermittent hormonal therapy	Continuous hormonal therapy	Metastatic prostate cancer	Hussain et al., 2013	• 1535 men randomized to intermittent versus continuous hormone therapy • At median follow-up of 9.8 years, survival was 5.1 years in the intermittent group and 5.8 years in the continuous group (HR 1.1 [0.99–1.23]) • Intermittent: significant improvements in mental function and erectile function

Seidenfeld J et al. *Ann Internal Med* 2000;132:566–77. [Prostate Cancer Trialists' Collaborative Group]. *Lancet* 2000;355:1491–8. [The Medical Research Council Prostate Cancer Working Party Investigators Group]. *Br J Urol* 1997;79:235–46. Messing EM et al. *Lancet Oncol* 2006;7:472–9. Crook JM et al. *N Engl J Med* 2012;367:895–903. Hussain M et al. *N Engl J Med* 2013;368:1314–25.
HR, hazard ratio; LHRH, luteinizing hormone-releasing hormone.

Key points – management of metastatic prostate cancer

- Treatment of metastatic prostate cancer is usually by androgen ablation.
- A luteinizing hormone-releasing hormone (LHRH) analog preceded and then accompanied by an antiandrogen is the most frequently employed treatment strategy.
- Treatment with a pure LHRH antagonist is another option, which avoids the need for an antiandrogen.
- Responses in terms of PSA reduction and clinical improvement are seen in more than 80% of patients.
- Eventually, however, androgen-insensitive cell clones develop and the PSA level begins to rise (castrate resistance).
- Side effects of medical castration include hot flashes, loss of libido and erectile dysfunction. The reduced testosterone levels are also associated with all the features of the metabolic syndrome.

Key references

Also see Table 7.4

Calais da Silva FE, Bono AV, Whelan P et al. Intermittent androgen deprivation for locally advanced and metastatic prostate cancer: results from a randomised phase 3 study of the South European Uroncological Group. *Eur Urol* 2009;55:1269–77.

Denis LD, Carneiro de Moura JL, Bono A et al. Goserelin acetate and flutamide versus bilateral orchidectomy: a phase III EORTC trial (30853). *Urology* 1993;42: 119–29.

Holmes-Walker DJ, Woo H, Gurney H et al. Maintaining bone health in patients with prostate cancer. *Med J Aust* 2006;184:176–9.

Klotz L, Boccon-Gibod L, Shore ND et al. The efficacy and safety of degarelix: a 12 month, comparative randomised, open-label, parallel-group phase III study in prostate cancer patients. *BJU Int* 2008;102:1531–8.

Langenhuijsen J, Schasfoort E, Heathcote P et al. Intermittent androgen suppression in patients with advanced prostate cancer: an update of the TULP survival data. *Eur Urol (suppl)* 2008;7:205, abstr 538.

Mittan D, Lee S, Miller E et al. Bone loss following hypogonadism in men with prostate cancer treated with GnRH analogs. *J Clin Endocrinol Metab* 2002;87:3656–61.

Prostate Cancer Trialists' Collaborative Group. Maximum androgen blockade in advanced prostate cancer: an overview of 22 randomized trials with 3283 deaths in 5710 patients. *Lancet* 1995;346:265–9.

Prostate Cancer Trialists' Collaborative Group. Maximum androgen blockade in advanced prostate cancer: an overview of the randomised trials. *Lancet* 2000;355:1491–8.

Tombal B, Miller K, Boccon-Gibod L et al. Additional analysis of the secondary end point of biochemical recurrence rate in a phase 3 trial (CS21) comparing degarelix 80 mg versus leuprolide in prostate cancer patients segmented by baseline characteristics. *Eur Urol* 2010;57:836–42.

Trachtenberg J, Gittleman M, Steidle C et al. A phase 3, multicenter, open label, randomized study of abarelix versus leuprolide plus daily antiandrogen in men with prostate cancer. *J Urol* 2002;167:1670–4.

8 Management of castrate-resistant prostate cancer

In most cases, advanced prostate cancers treated with any form of androgen-deprivation therapy (ADT) eventually begin to progress, a phenomenon known as 'castrate resistance'. An increase in PSA level after initially successful androgen deprivation almost inevitably indicates impending clinical progression. Castrate-resistant prostate cancer (CRPC) has been characterized as disease that has progressed despite the persistence of castrate levels of androgens (< 1.73 nmol/L or 50 ng/dL), but remains hormone sensitive and is amenable to further hormonal manipulations. This state probably arises from either clonal selection of androgen-independent cell lines (Figure 8.1) or increased ligand-independent activation of androgen receptors.

Men with CRPC are quite a heterogeneous group; they include men with increasing PSA only and no demonstrable metastases, and men who have many bone and/or visceral metastases (Figure 8.2), pain and poor functional status. Survival can range from only a few months to 4 years or more. Historically, therapy had little effect beyond modest

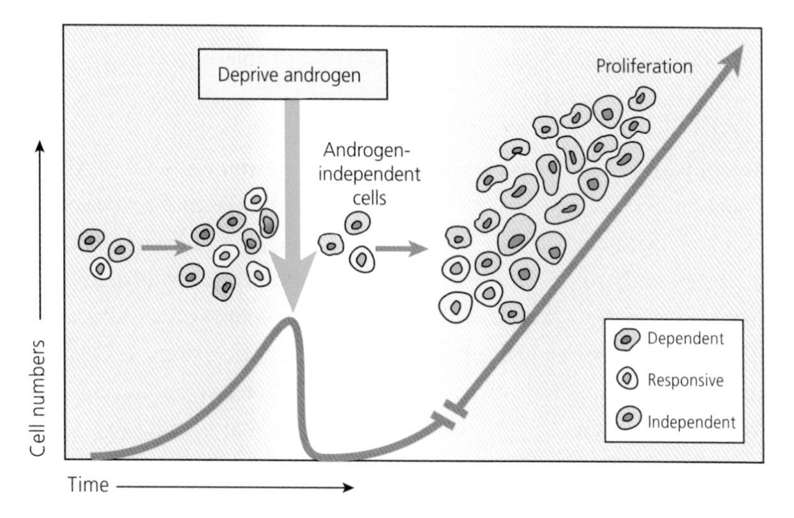

Figure 8.1 Hormone escape results from selection of castrate-resistant cells.

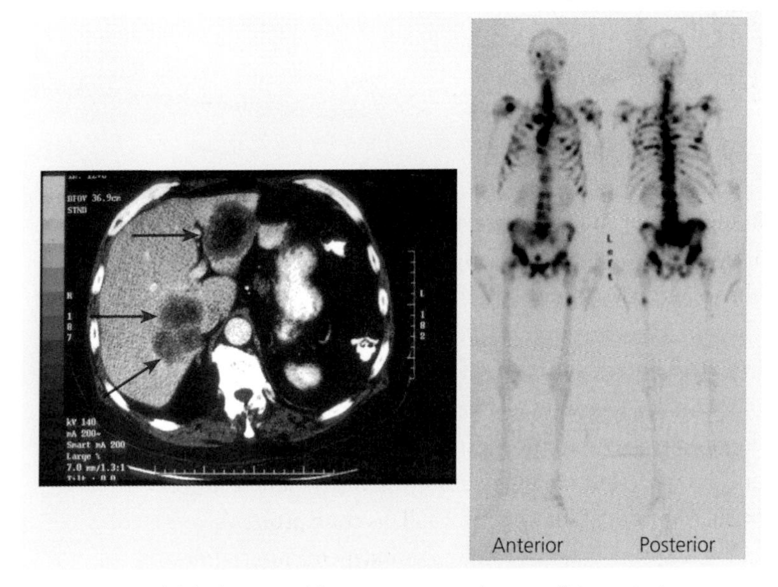

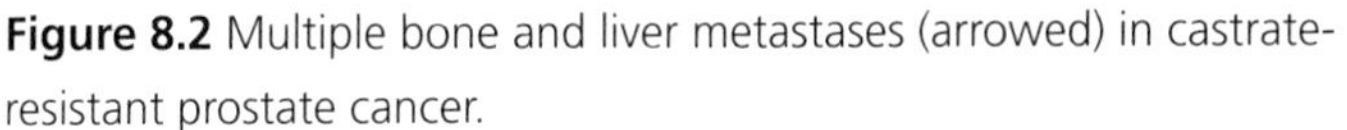

Figure 8.2 Multiple bone and liver metastases (arrowed) in castrate-resistant prostate cancer.

palliation. More recently, significantly more options have become available and there are now several treatments that not only improve quality of life and pain palliation, but also increase survival (Figure 8.3).

Some of the trials with important results for the treatment of CRPC are summarized at the end of this chapter (see Table 8.1).

Further hormonal manipulation

Antiandrogens. When the serum PSA level rises after a period of ADT alone, an initial move may be to add an antiandrogen to the treatment. This may transiently reduce PSA, but the PSA will usually start to rise again relatively soon. At this time, withdrawal of the antiandrogen may also produce a favorable PSA response (in approximately 40% of men) for 4–6 months. This phenomenon (which also occurs in breast cancer treated with antiestrogens) has been ascribed to a mutation affecting androgen receptors in malignant tissue that means the antiandrogen acts as an agonist (stimulatory) rather than an antagonist (blocker), so when the antiandrogen is withdrawn the stimulation is reduced. As long as the patient is asymptomatic, the

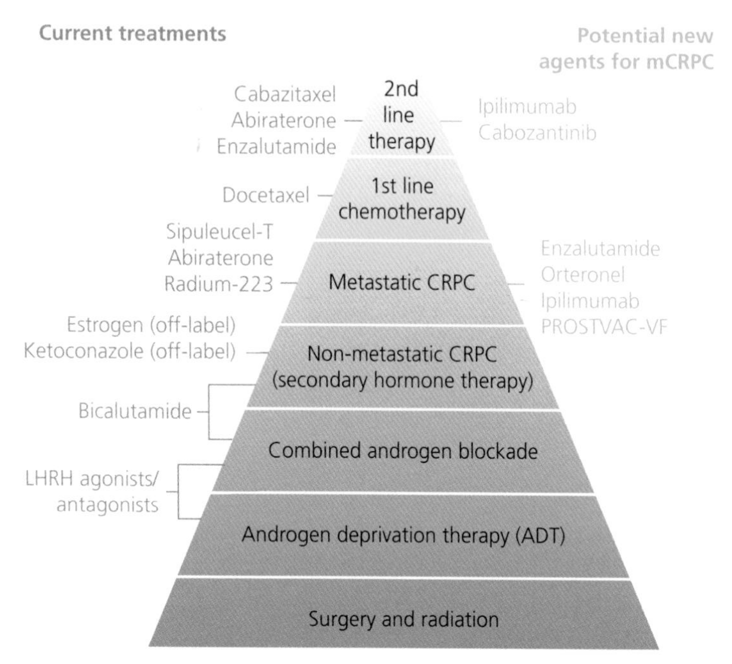

Figure 8.3 Established, newly available and potential treatments for castrate-resistant prostate cancer (CRPC). Adapted from Shore et al., 2012. LHRH, luteinizing hormone-releasing hormone.

addition and withdrawal of different antiandrogens can be continued for two to three cycles, as previous antiandrogen administration does not appear to diminish the response to different antiandrogens.

Adrenal androgen synthesis inhibitors. In addition to antiandrogens, research has shown that antiandrogen withdrawal followed by inhibitors of adrenal androgen synthesis, such as aminoglutethimide or ketoconazole, results in good reductions in PSA levels. However, adrenal androgen synthesis inhibitors are very toxic and not well tolerated, so this is not a usual treatment option.

Estrogen treatment may benefit some men with CRPC. It appears to have two effects:

- inhibition of pituitary gonadotropin secretion
- direct cytotoxic effect on the tumor.

The synthetic estrogen diethylstilbestrol (DES) has been used in prostate cancer, but its use as first-line therapy is limited by side effects such as gynecomastia, deep-vein thrombosis and other cardiovascular complications. A combination of DES with acetylsalicylic acid (ASA; aspirin) or warfarin may reduce the thrombotic and cardiovascular toxicity that can be very hazardous in men of this age, but patients should be alerted to the risks.

Non-metastatic (M0) castrate-resistant prostate cancer

Men who start ADT before any metastases are demonstrated, such as for a rising PSA after radiotherapy, may become castrate resistant without any evidence of distant metastases (M0 CRPC). These men can present a difficult management dilemma, because although they are asymptomatic their rising PSA can cause significant psychological distress.

Traditionally, treatment has been either further hormonal manipulations as described above or treatment administered as part of a clinical trial. Once these fail, however, an observational approach is taken until the patient develops demonstrable metastases (M1 CRPC) for which further treatments are available (see below).

A number of therapies, such as the endothelin antagonists atrasenten and zibotentan (ZD4054), have been trialed to determine if the onset of M1 CRPC can be delayed. To date, no therapy has been effective in delaying the progression of M0 CRPC to M1 CRPC. A plethora of new drugs are being evaluated and, with time, it is possible that one or more may be effective for this disease stage.

Metastatic (M1) castrate-resistant prostate cancer

Abiraterone is approved as first-line treatment for metastatic CRPC. It is a specific inhibitor of cytochrome P450 17-hydroxylase/17,20-lyase (CYP17), a key enzyme in androgen synthesis (Figure 8.4). Abiraterone is effective in CRPC because, despite castrate levels of circulating androgens from luteinizing hormone-releasing hormone (LHRH) agonist therapy, CRPC cells have been shown to synthesize their own androgens from cholesterol, which then perpetuate androgen receptor signaling. In a randomized trial involving 1088 men

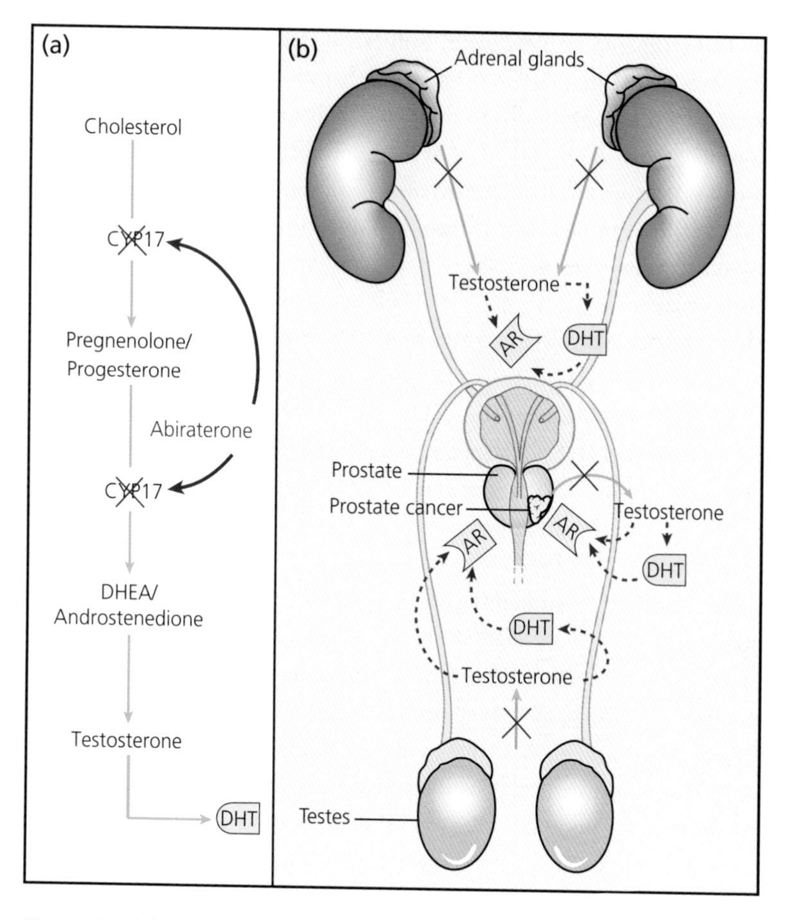

Figure 8.4 (a) Androgen biosynthesis. By inhibiting the action of cytochrome P450 17-hydroxylase/17,20-lyase (CYP17) – a key enzyme in the biosynthesis of androgens from cholesterol – abiraterone interferes with the production of dehydroepiandrosterone (DHEA) and androstenedione, precursors of testosterone and dihydrotestosterone (DHT). (b) While castration leads to decreased production of testosterone and DHT by the testes, the adrenal glands and prostate cancer tissue continue to produce these androgens, leading to activation of androgen receptors (ARs) and continued prostate cancer growth. Abiraterone blocks the production of testosterone and DHT via the pathway shown in (a) at all three of these sites, thus providing an alternative treatment for patients with castrate-resistant prostate cancer.

with asymptomatic or mildly symptomatic metastatic CRPC who had not received previous chemotherapy, abiraterone plus prednisone improved radiographic progression-free survival and overall survival compared with prednisone only and delayed PSA progression and the times to opiate use and initiation of cytotoxic chemotherapy (see Table 8.1). The incidence of grade 3/4 mineralocorticoid-related adverse events and liver-function abnormalities was higher in the group receiving abiraterone, but no unique toxic events occurred with abiraterone treatment.

Docetaxel, a member of the taxoid family, induces apoptosis in cells through microtubule stabilization. It has been established as first-line therapy for men with M1 CRPC for many years. A randomized trial (TAX-327) comparing docetaxel with mitoxantrone (another chemotherapy drug) and prednisone in men with CRPC found that a 3-week schedule of docetaxel was superior to mitoxantrone/prednisone in terms of disease progression and overall survival (see Table 8.1). In this trial, the incidence of neutropenia, skin reactions and gastrointestinal problems was higher in the group receiving docetaxel than in the group receiving the mitoxantrone/prednisone combination. These are the most common side effects with docetaxel, but in general the chemotherapeutic agent is well tolerated.

Second-line therapy. When prostate cancer progresses after docetaxel chemotherapy, a number of options for further treatment exist, including further chemotherapy or one of the new hormonal modulation agents.

Cabazitaxel. This taxane chemotherapy was developed to overcome the resistance that can develop as a result of docetaxel treatment. The TROPIC study randomized men with CRPC who had progressed after docetaxel treatment to cabazitaxel or mitoxantrone chemotherapy. Participants receiving cabazitaxel demonstrated a 30% improvement in survival (15.1 months versus 12.7 months, compared with those receiving mitoxantrone; Figure 8.5 and see Table 8.1). Side effects are similar to those seen with docetaxel.

Mitoxantrone and prednisone was the first chemotherapy combination to be tested in a randomized fashion in advanced prostate

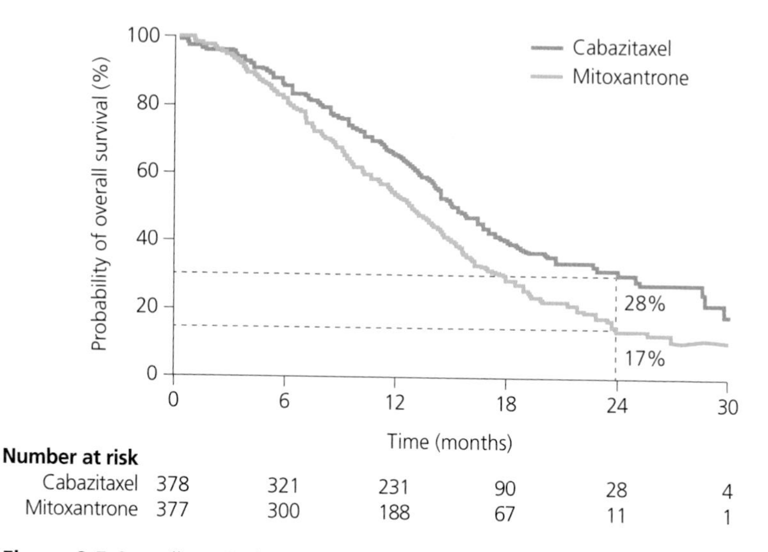

Figure 8.5 Overall survival in the TROPIC trial. At 2 years, 28% of patients in the cabazitaxel group were alive compared with 17% in the mitoxantrone group. From de Bono JS et al. *Lancet* 2010;376:1147–54, reproduced with permission from Elsevier.

cancer. The trial showed that this combination was very well tolerated and more than doubled the time of palliation response when compared with prednisone alone. It also improved the quality of life of men with CRPC. It has been replaced by docetaxel as first-line chemotherapy and cabazitaxel as second-line chemotherapy because of inferior efficacy. This combination still has a limited place in second-line therapy when resistance to docetaxel has developed and cabazitaxel is not an option for therapy.

Abiraterone. In a study of abiraterone plus prednisone in men with metastatic CRPC for whom docetaxel chemotherapy had failed abiraterone plus prednisone resulted in a 35% improvement in survival compared with prednisone alone (see Table 8.1). Mineralocorticoid-related adverse events, including fluid retention, hypertension and hypokalemia, were more frequently reported in the abiraterone group than in the control group, highlighting the continuing dependency of CRPC on androgen-receptor signaling, even after the cancer has become castrate resistant (see Table 8.1).

Orteronel (TAK-700), like abiraterone, is another orally active, selective inhibitor of 17,20-lyase. It is currently being investigated in phase III trials. However, a recent trial was unblinded after an interim analysis indicated that the combination of orteronel and prednisone was not likely to meet the primary endpoint of improved overall survival compared with a control arm of placebo and prednisone in men with metastatic CRPC that had progressed during or after chemotherapy. Other studies looking at the addition of orteronel in chemotherapy-naïve patients are ongoing.

Enzalutamide (formerly MDV3100) is an androgen-receptor-signaling inhibitor, approved for the treatment of patients with metastatic CRPC who have previously been treated with docetaxel. It inhibits nuclear translocation of the androgen receptor, DNA binding and coactivator recruitment (Figure 8.6). It also has a greater affinity for the receptor than non-steroidal antiandrogens and no known agonistic effects. In the AFFIRM randomized controlled trial, oral enzalutamide, 160 mg/day, improved survival in men with metastatic CRPC after docetaxel chemotherapy (see Table 8.1). However, rates of fatigue, diarrhea and hot flashes were higher in the enzalutamide group.

The PREVAIL trial is currently investigating the efficacy of enzalutamide in men with metastatic CRPC prior to chemotherapy.

Immunotherapy

Therapies involving modulation of the immune system are showing considerable promise in trials of CRPC. These therapies, however, do take time to mediate an effect and are best used in men with minimal or no symptoms.

Sipuleucel-T is an autologous cellular immunotherapy. In a phase III trial of men with CRPC not yet treated with docetaxel, treatment with sipuleucel-T resulted in a 22% relative reduction in the risk of death compared with placebo, with minimal treatment side effects (see Table 8.1). This is the first immunotherapy in prostate cancer that has demonstrated a survival advantage. Treatment is, however, complicated and requires a specialized laboratory, which makes it extremely expensive to administer.

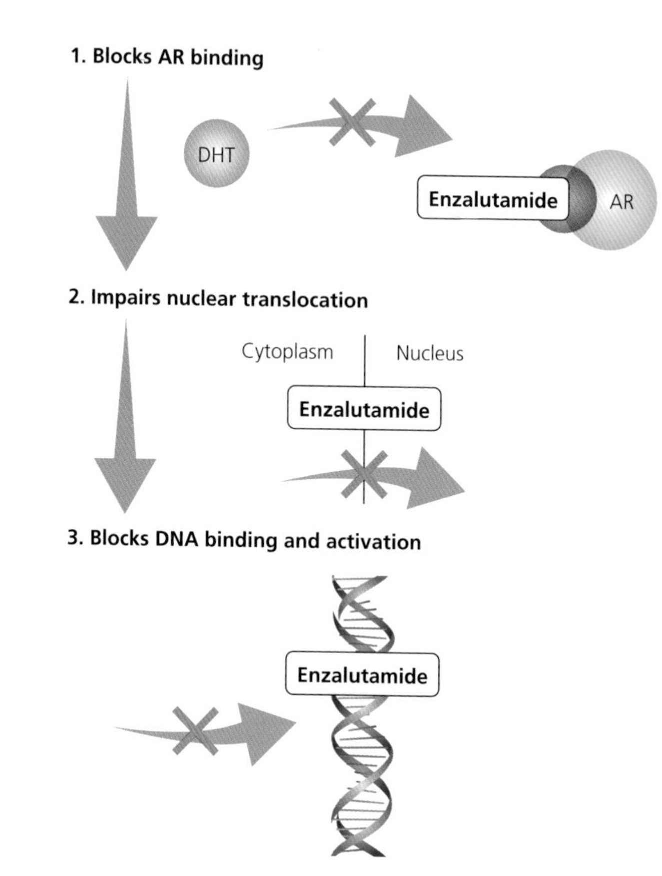

Figure 8.6 Mechanism of action of enzalutamide, which inhibits androgen receptor signaling in three ways. Based on Tran C et al. Science 2009;324:787–90; and Watson PA et al. *Proc Natl Acad Sci USA* 2010;107:16759–65. AR, androgen receptor; DHT, dihydrotestosterone.

Ipilimumab. Cytotoxic T-lymphocyte antigen-4 (CTLA-4), which is a negative regulator of T-cell activation, has emerged as a target for cancer immunotherapy. Ipilimumab, a fully human monoclonal antibody, specifically blocks the binding of CTLA-4 to its ligands and thereby augments T-cell activation and proliferation resulting in tumor regression. Significant tumor responses with ipilimumab were identified in a phase II trial in men with metastatic CRPC. This immunotherapy is currently in phase III trials.

PROSTVAC-VF is a prostate cancer vaccine regimen consisting of a recombinant vaccinia vector as a primary vaccination, followed by multiple booster vaccinations employing a recombinant fowlpox vector. These vaccines stimulate an antigen presenting cell-mediated immune response to PSA-expressing tumor cells. In a small randomized study of men with metastatic CRPC, those treated with PROSTVAC-VF had better overall survival compared with the placebo group (25.1 months vs 16.6 months). These results are promising but need confirmation in larger randomized trials.

Management of bone metastases

Bone pain is one of the most intractable problems associated with CRPC, and conventional analgesics may not always provide relief.

Palliative radiotherapy. Men with hormone-naïve disease will initially be managed by ADT. However, some men will not get full pain resolution or may have painful bone metastases in the setting of CRPC.

Focal external-beam radiotherapy is a well-established treatment, and up to 80% of treated men experience rapid improvement in pain. Treatment can be given as a single fraction or as multiple fractions over 2–3 weeks. There are very few side effects associated with this type of irradiation.

Wide-field radiation may also be useful in patients with intractable diffuse pain. This treatment can delay the progression of existing disease as well as slow the occurrence of new disease, but it produces side effects such as pneumonitis, cataracts, nausea, vomiting and diarrhea in approximately 35% of patients, and severe, sometimes irreversible, hematological effects in 9%.

Systemic radionuclide therapy is a means of targeting multiple painful bone metastases by intravenously administering a radionuclide (such as samarium-153) complexed to bone-avid molecules such as ethylene diamine tetra (methylene phosphonic acid) (EDTMP), or radionuclides that have a natural affinity to metabolically active bone, such as strontium-89. After administration of samarium-153, 65–80% of patients report relief from pain and symptoms within 1 week. The average duration of response is 2–3 months. The major toxicity is myelosuppression, which can last a number of months – white blood cell count and platelet levels should be monitored before and after therapy.

Radium-223 is a bone-seeking radionucleotide that delivers local radiotherapy by emitting alpha radiation. As alpha particles have limited penetration, radium-223 delivers highly localized therapy, killing tumor cells with minimal damage to surrounding tissue. In the phase III ALSYMPCA study, which involved patients with CRPC and bone metastases who had failed or were unsuitable for docetaxel treatment, radium-223 with best supportive care was compared with placebo. Overall survival was improved with the radionucleotide (see Table 8.1). Side effects of radium-223 include increased low-grade nausea, diarrhea and occasional neutropenia. It is approved for the treatment of patients with CRPC, symptomatic bone metastases and no known visceral metastatic disease.

Bisphosphonates. Some patients benefit symptomatically from treatment with bisphosphonates, which suppress bone resorption and demineralization. A study involving over 600 patients with CRPC that compared zoledronic acid (zoledronate), given as an intravenous infusion every 3 weeks, with placebo demonstrated a significant reduction in the number of patients with bone-related events in those receiving zoledronic acid. It also significantly delayed the onset of first bone-related event (see Table 8.1). It would, however, require ten men to be treated to save one from a bone-related event. Side effects with bisphosphonates include renal deterioration and, rarely, jaw necrosis.

Denosumab is a human monoclonal antibody directed against the receptor activator of nuclear factor κ-B ligand (RANKL). It inhibits osteoclast function and bone turnover. Findings from a randomized trial involving 1904 men with CRPC support denosumab as the optimal medication to reduce bone-related events in men with CRPC (see Table 8.1).

Palliative care

Despite improving therapies, most patients with CRPC eventually die as a result of the cancer, often within 12–24 months. Treatment with high-dose steroids can sometimes provide useful palliation. The palliative care of these patients requires a supportive and caring team approach involving the family physician, the urologist, an experienced palliative care team and, of course, the patient's close relatives and friends.

Treatment algorithm

A suggested algorithm for treatment is given in Figure 8.7.

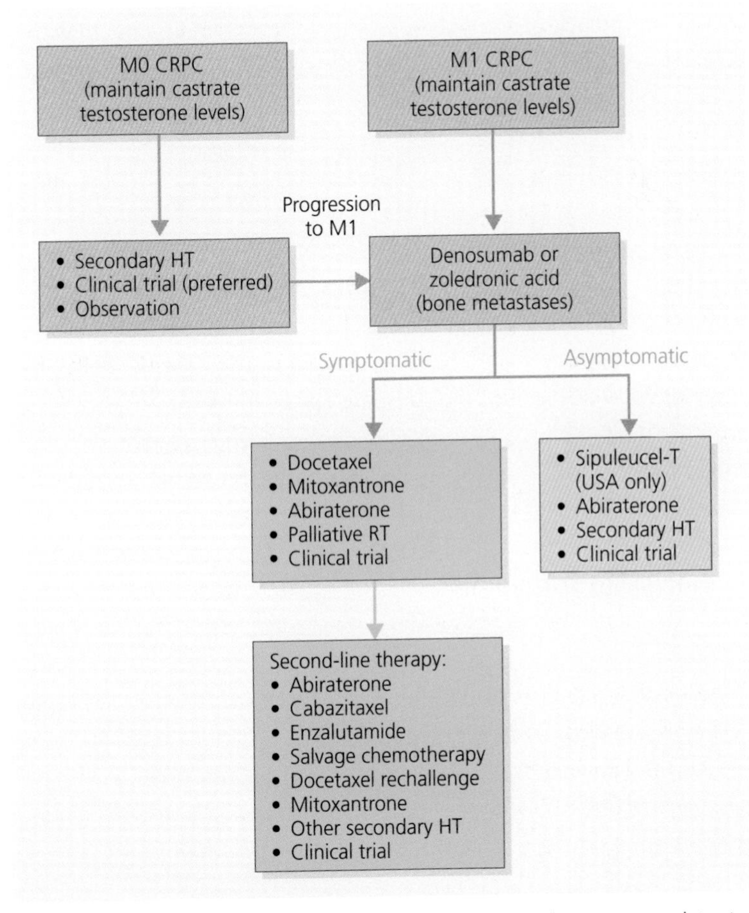

Figure 8.7 Suggested treatment algorithm for men with castrate-resistant prostate cancer (CRPC). Adapted from Shore et al., 2012. HT, hormone therapy; RT, radiotherapy.

TABLE 8.1

Important trials in the treatment of castrate-resistant prostate cancer

Medication	Use	Trial	Key outcomes
Docetaxel (chemotherapy), 3-weekly schedule	First-line M1 CRPC	Tannock et al., 2004 (TAX-327)	Versus mitoxantrone plus prednisone, 1006 men randomized: • decreased disease progression and PSA response • increased pain improvement and quality of life • improved survival (18.9 versus 16.4 months; 24% relative reduction in death) • increased incidence of neutropenia, skin reactions and GI problems
Cabazitaxel (chemotherapy)	Second-line M1 CRPC	de Bono et al., 2010 (TROPIC)	Versus mitoxantrone, 755 men randomized: • improved survival (15.1 months versus 12.7 months), 30% RR in deaths • neutropenia and diarrhea were the most common side effects
Mitoxantrone plus prednisone (chemotherapy)	First-line M1 CRPC	Tannock et al., 1996	Versus prednisone, 161 men randomized: • no difference in survival observed • significant improvement in palliative response and quality of life

CONTINUED

TABLE 8.1 (CONTINUED)

Medication	Use	Trial	Key outcomes
Abiraterone plus prednisone (AR targeted)	M1 CRPC before chemotherapy	Ryan et al., 2013	Versus placebo plus prednisone, 1088 men randomized: • improved progression-free survival (16.5 months versus 8.3 months), RR for death 47% • improved overall survival (median not reached versus 27.2 months), RR for death 25% • delayed the initiation of chemotherapy
Abiraterone plus prednisone (AR targeted)	Following docetaxel chemotherapy in M1 CRPC	de Bono et al., 2011	Versus placebo plus prednisone, 1195 men randomized 2:1 • increased survival 14.8 months versus 10.9 months, RR for death 35% • mineralocorticoid-related adverse events, including fluid retention, hypertension and hypokalemia
Enzalutamide (AR targeted)	Following docetaxel chemotherapy in M1 CRPC	Scher et al., 2012 (AFFIRM)	Versus placebo, 1199 men randomized • improved overall survival (18.4 months versus 13.6 months), RR for death 37% • improvements in PSA response, soft tissue response, quality of life and time to first skeletal-related event • side effects of fatigue, diarrhea and hot flashes as well as, rarely, seizures

CONTINUED

TABLE 8.1 (CONTINUED)

Medication	Use	Trial	Key outcomes
Sipuleucel-T (immunotherapy)	M1 CRPC	Kantoff et al., 2010	Versus placebo, 512 men randomized • improved survival (25.8 months versus 21.7 months), RR for death 22% • treatment side effects were minimal
Radium-223 (radio-isotope)	M1 CRPC	Parker et al., 2013 (ALSYMPCA)	Versus placebo, 921 men randomized • improved overall survival (14.0 months versus 11.2 months), RR for death 30% • associated with low myelosuppression rates and fewer adverse events
Zoledronic acid (bisphosphonate)	M1 CRPC	Saad et al., 2002	Doses 4 mg versus 8 mg versus placebo, 643 men randomized 1:1:1 • median time to first skeletal-related event increased in 4 mg dose versus 8 mg versus placebo (not reached versus 363 days versus 321days) • pain and analgesic scores were higher in placebo group
Denosumab (monoclonal antibody)	M1 CRPC	Fizazi et al., 2011	Versus zoledronic acid, 1904 men randomized • increased median time to first skeletal-related event (20.7 months versus 17.1 months), HR 0.82 • adverse events were equivalent in both arms

Tannock IF et al. *N Engl J Med* 2004;351:1502–12. de Bono JS et al. *Lancet* 2010;376:1147–54. Tannock IF et al. *J Clin Oncol* 1996;14:1756–64. Ryan CJ et al. *N Engl J Med* 2013;368:138–48. de Bono JS et al. *N Engl J Med* 2011;364:1995–2005. Scher HI et al. *N Engl J Med* 2012;367:1187–97. Kantoff PW et al. *N Engl J Med* 2010;363:411–22. Parker C et al. *N Engl J Med* 2013;369:213–23. Saad F et al. *J Natl Cancer Inst* 2002;94:1458–68. Fizazi K et al. *Lancet* 2011;377:813–22.

AR, androgen receptor; CRPC, castrate-resistant prostate cancer; GI, gastrointestinal; HR, hazard ratio; PSA, prostate-specific antigen; RR, relative risk.

Key points – management of castrate-resistant prostate cancer

- After an initial response to androgen ablation, the serum PSA value starts to rise as a result of androgen-insensitive cell clones.
- As an initial maneuver, withdraw any antiandrogen the patient is taking, then consider trying another antiandrogen.
- The mainstay of management for metastatic castrate-resistant prostate cancer (CRPC) is treatment with docetaxel chemotherapy. However, the CYP17 inhibitor abiraterone is now licensed for use before chemotherapy, and trials of other antiandrogens prior to chemotherapy are under way.
- When docetaxel chemotherapy has failed, second-line therapies such as cabazitaxel chemotherapy, abiraterone (a selective inhibitor of androgen biosynthesis) and enzalutamide (an androgen-receptor-signaling inhibitor) have all been shown to improve survival and quality of life.
- Immunotherapy for CRPC may be best implemented before men have significant symptoms.
- The monoclonal antibody denosumab and the bisphosphonate zoledronic acid have been reported to delay significantly bone-related events in men with metastatic prostate cancer.
- External-beam radiotherapy may provide useful control of pain from bone metastases.
- Radium-223 seems a promising new treatment for bone metastases.

Key references

Also see Table 8.1

Fizazi K, Scher HI, Molina A et al. Abiraterone acetate for treatment of metastatic castration-resistant prostate cancer: final overall survival analysis of the COU-AA-301 randomised, double-blind, placebo-controlled phase 3 study. *Lancet Oncol* 2012;13:983–92.

Kantoff PW, Schuetz TJ, Blumenstein BA et al. Overall survival analysis of a phase II randomized controlled trial of a Poxviral-based PSA-targeted immunotherapy in metastatic castration-resistant prostate cancer. *J Clin Oncol* 2010;28:1099–105.

Lewington VJ, McEwan AJ, Ackery DM et al. A prospective, randomised double-blind crossover study to examine the efficacy of strontium-89 in pain palliation in patients with advanced prostate cancer metastatic to bone. *Eur J Cancer* 1991;27:954–8.

National Institute for Health and Care Excellence. Abiraterone for castration-resistant metastatic prostate cancer previously treated with a docetaxel-containing regimen. NICE Technology Appraisal No. 259. June 2012. http://guidance.nice.org.uk/TA259, last accessed 22 October 2013.

Scher HI, Fizazi K, Saad F et al. Increased survival with enzalutamide in prostate cancer after chemotherapy. *N Engl J Med* 2012;367:1187–97.

Scher HI, Kelly WK. Flutamide withdrawal syndrome: its impact on clinical trials in hormone-refractory prostate cancer. *J Clin Oncol* 1993;11:1566–72.

Shore N, Mason M. de Reijke TM. New developments in castrate-resistant prostate cancer. *BJU Int* 2012;109(Suppl6):22–32.

Slovin SF, Higano CS, Hamid O et al. Ipilimumab alone or in combination with radiotherapy in metastatic castration-resistant prostate cancer: results from an open-label, multicenter phase I/II study. *Ann Oncol* 2013;24:1813–21.

Smith MR, Egerdie B, Hernandez Toriz N et al. Denosumab in men receiving androgen-deprivation therapy for prostate cancer. *N Engl J Med* 2009;361:745–55.

9 Survivorship and treatment complications

With more and more men with prostate cancer surviving for longer and longer, 'survivorship' issues are becoming increasingly important. Primary care practitioners and allied healthcare professionals have an important role here: good management of treatment effects and complications can unquestionably improve the quality of life of affected men and should be incorporated into the routine care of all prostate cancer survivors. Remember, survivorship years can be some of the best years your patients have.

With this in mind, survivorship is not only about treating, but also supporting, the whole individual, as well as his immediate family, throughout the entire cancer journey. Psychological issues as well as medical matters need to be managed, including anxiety related to the cancer and its cure, depression, and fear of recurrence after treatment. In this respect those who care for men with prostate cancer could learn a great deal from the teams and charities that treat and support those with breast cancer.

Other healthcare professionals, especially urology nurse specialists, have a crucial role in encouraging prostate cancer survivors to share their concerns with loved ones, treatment teams, mental health professionals and prostate cancer support groups, as well as fellow survivors. Nurses also have a key role in referral of patients to the most appropriate advisory and support services.

Sexual function

A diagnosis of prostate cancer alone may be enough to disturb sex lives that, in the age group usually affected, are sometimes already beginning to wane.

Erectile dysfunction. Treatment of localized prostate cancer often results in sexual dysfunction. Erectile dysfunction is the most common complaint and can occur after all treatments. Improvements in techniques for radical prostatectomy and nerve sparing, such as the use of robotic assistance, have resulted in very significant improvements in this area; however, erectile dysfunction can occur following even the most expert surgery. Unfortunately, it is also sometimes necessary to deliberately resect the cavernous nerves in order to resect widely to avoid positive surgical margins. Obviously this can have detrimental effects on erectile function.

Limited success regarding erectile function has been reported for the replacement of resected nerves with sural nerve grafts after surgery (Figure 9.1).

Intracorporeal fibrosis results from the release of transforming growth factor α (TGFα). As TGFα is released in response to anoxia, therapies that bring oxygenated arterial blood into the corpora and induce erection inhibit its release and may help maintain smooth muscle function. Early administration of pharmaceutical treatments for erectile dysfunction soon after surgery has been shown to improve the time and quality of subsequent erections. Montorsi et al. have shown in a randomized trial that early intracavernosal injections with alprostadil (prostaglandin E_1), once or twice a week, result in early recovery of spontaneous erections after nerve-sparing radical

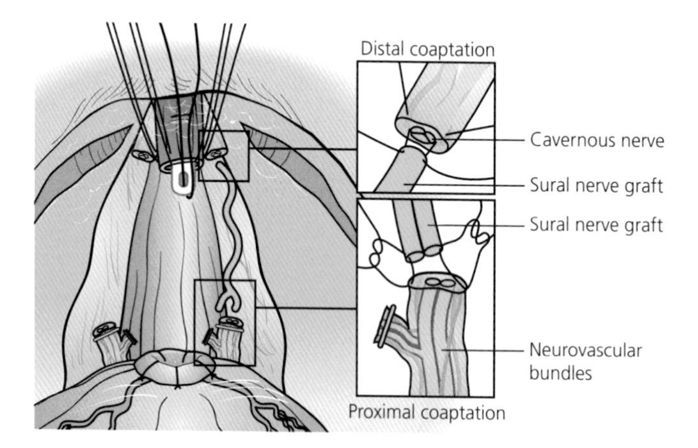

Figure 9.1 Sural nerve graft interposition to restore erectile function following prostatectomy.

prostatectomy. Early administration of phosphodiesterase type 5 (PDE5) inhibitors, such as tadalafil, 5 mg daily, has also been shown to improve the time and quality of spontaneous erections after bilateral nerve-sparing surgery. Patients refractory to intracavernosal and oral PDE5 inhibitor treatment have the option of using a vacuum constriction device to obtain erections or surgery to insert an inflatable penile prosthesis (Figure 9.2).

External-beam radiotherapy and brachytherapy are both associated with an incidence of delayed-onset erectile dysfunction of 30% or more. Cryotherapy very often results in erectile dysfunction because the neurovascular bundles are included in the freezing zone. Similarly, high-intensity focused ultrasound (HIFU) can result in impaired erectile function if the neurovascular bundles are in the treated area. Treatment is along the same lines as that for erectile dysfunction following prostatectomy (see also *Fast Facts: Erectile Dysfunction*).

Ejaculatory problems. Men undergoing treatment for localized prostate cancer by radical prostatectomy or transurethral resection of the prostate (TURP) may also experience ejaculatory problems, though sensation of orgasm is usually preserved. In the case of TURP, semen

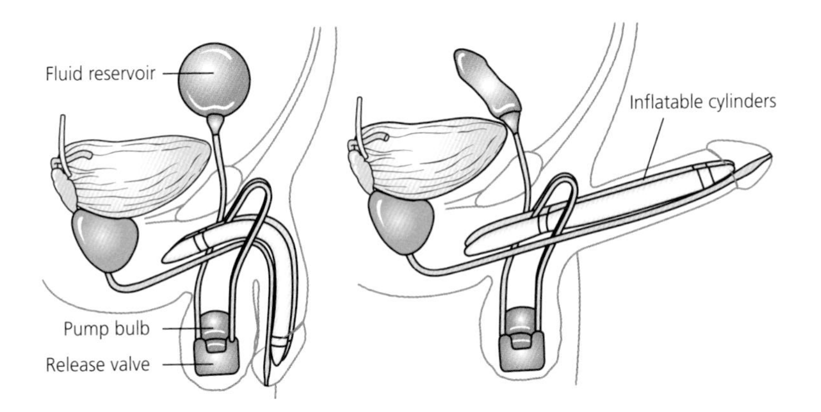

Figure 9.2 An inflatable penile prosthesis. Squeezing the pump transfers fluid from the reservoir into the cylinders, causing an erection. Pushing the release valve drains the fluid back to the abdominal reservoir.

is still produced, but it passes retrogradely into the bladder. After radical prostatectomy, in which the entire prostate and seminal vesicles have been removed, no semen is produced, but most patients are still able to achieve orgasm. Patients must be informed about these consequences before surgery. Drugs such as the α_1-blocker tamsulosin, used to treat bladder outflow obstruction, may also cause loss of, or reduced, ejaculation, but this is reversible on cessation of treatment.

Loss of libido is a common complaint of patients with prostate cancer. It may result from the disease itself causing debilitation or depression. More commonly, it is a side effect of hormone ablation therapy. Bilateral orchidectomy or therapy with luteinizing hormone-releasing hormone (LHRH) analogs or pure LHRH antagonists is almost invariably associated with loss of libido, as well as erectile dysfunction. Therapy with an antiandrogen can effectively deprive prostate cancer cells of androgen stimulation without such a profound effect on libido or erectile function.

Preservation of sexual function. If this is an important factor in terms of the quality of life of the individual with prostate cancer, then treatment with an antiandrogen as monotherapy may well be considered as an alternative to bilateral orchidectomy or an LHRH analog.

Counseling. The most important conclusion to be drawn is that patients with prostate cancer, as well as their partners, should be counseled not only about probable outcomes, but also about the likely effect of the disease and its therapy on their sex lives. A more open and informed approach to this important aspect of prostate cancer will do much not only to counter the anxiety and loss of self-esteem that so often accompany the diagnosis of this prevalent malignancy, but also to restore effective sexual function after treatment and thereby maintain an important aspect of quality of life.

Urinary and bowel symptoms

Incontinence following radical prostatectomy. Radical prostatectomy involves removing the prostate gland and some of the bladder neck.

The contribution of the bladder neck and prostatic smooth muscle to normal continence is lost following surgery. Operative injury to the remaining rhabdosphincter or its nerve supply is probably the most common factor in post-prostatectomy incontinence. Other factors that may contribute are bladder instability, which may have existed before surgery or developed after, and a poorly compliant bladder. Following removal of the urethral catheter after surgery, some degree of immediate stress incontinence is expected, followed by gradual improvement in urinary control. Factors that contribute to the early recovery of continence are:

- younger age of the patient
- experienced surgeon
- bilateral nerve-sparing surgery
- absence of anastamotic stricture
- performing pelvic floor exercises before and following surgery.

Treatment is initially conservative, with control of fluid intake and pelvic floor exercises. Treatment of bladder instability involves anticholinergic medication. If this fails, options include injection of peri-urethral bulking agent, which has approximately 40% success in the short term. Other options are the insertion of a bulbo-urethral sling or artificial urinary sphincter (see *Fast Facts: Bladder Disorders*).

Urinary and bowel symptoms from radiotherapy. During the delivery of radiotherapy, irritative symptoms of urgency and frequency are very common, being considerably worse with high-dose-rate (HDR) brachytherapy and seed brachytherapy than with external-beam radiotherapy. They tend to settle with time, however. Later urinary symptoms can comprise irritative symptoms such as urgency and frequency, pain and even incontinence and can be due to instability, poor compliance, urethral stricture, overflow incontinence, bladder ulcer or a combination of these.

Rectal symptoms may also be troublesome after radiotherapy. Diarrhea, tenesmus and rectal bleeding may all occur. These tend to resolve over time, but patients should be made aware that external-beam radiotherapy is associated with an increased risk of colorectal cancer. Persistent rectal bleeding should be investigated by colonoscopy.

Treatment is also initially conservative, and involves changes to lifestyle as well as identification of the cause and individualized treatment.

Adverse effects of hormonal therapy

Prospective clinical trials of androgen-deprivation therapy (ADT) for men with prostate cancer demonstrate the development of multiple risk factors for bone health and cardiovascular disease, including increases in serum cholesterol and triglycerides, insulin resistance, body mass index and fat body mass, together with decreases in lean body mass (Table 9.1).

Hot flashes, where a rise in the temperature of the face and trunk is accompanied by cutaneous vasodilatation – affecting mainly the face, throat and extremities – and sweating, are common in men using ADT. ADT-related hormone changes result in the release of catecholamines, notably norepinephrine (noradrenaline), from the hypothalamus, which interferes with thermoregulation controlled by the upper hypothalamus.

TABLE 9.1

Potential effects of androgen-deprivation therapy

Metabolic effects	Physical changes
• Hyperlipidemia	• Increased fat mass
• Insulin resistance and diabetes	• Decreased muscle mass
• Osteoporosis	• Loss of body hair
• Increased risk of fracture anemia	• Gynecomastia
	• Hot flashes
Mental changes	**Sexual effects**
• Decreased cognition	• Decreased libido
• Emotional changes	• Erectile dysfunction

Men should be counseled that hot flashes may continue despite efforts to overcome them, and advised to take steps to minimize the discomfort they can cause (for example, wearing lighter weight clothing). Some hormonal treatments, such as the α_2 receptor antagonist clonidine, may help, but all can have side effects that may outweigh the benefits. Progestins such as megestrol acetate seem to have the best side-effect profile. Other agents such as selective serotonin-reuptake inhibitors (SSRIs) may also be acceptable. There is currently little evidence to support the use of complementary therapies.

Fatigue and anemia. Fatigue resulting from hormone therapy is complex and overlaps with other side effects such as depression and pain. It can have a considerable impact on a man's quality of life as it may affect normal functioning and sleep.

Exercise and dietary advice constitute the first-line approach. Research has shown that following a regular exercise program can help overcome the weakness and muscle wasting that may develop with ADT, and reduce the frequency and severity of fatigue. Often the involvement of a dietitian and exercise physiologist can be beneficial.

There is a suggestion that intermittent ADT may be associated with lower fatigue than continuous ADT, but currently this is not supported by strong trial evidence.

Anemia tends to be worse with maximum androgen blockade with LHRH agonist/antiandrogen than with LHRH agonist or antiandrogen monotherapy. Hemoglobin levels rise slowly after treatment has ended. Newly diagnosed men should have a blood count before starting ADT to check for pretreatment anemia and vitamin B_{12}, folate or iron deficiencies. Hemoglobin levels should be monitored throughout ADT. Transfusions are recommended if hemoglobin is below 10 g/dL in symptomatic men and in asymptomatic men with comorbidities such as congestive heart failure or cerebral vascular disease.

Breast symptoms. Men may experience gynecomastia and mastalgia (swollen and painful breasts) while using some forms of ADT. The likelihood varies with treatment, with men using antiandrogens or estrogens having the highest risk.

In England and Wales, the National Institute for Health and Care Excellence (NICE) recommends prophylactic radiotherapy to both breast buds within the first month of long-term treatment with the antiandrogen bicalutamide (150 mg monotherapy for more than 6 months). While this makes sense as a palliative measure for men with advanced disease, for men with locally advanced disease, the pros and cons of prophylactic radiotherapy need careful consideration as there is a risk of a second malignancy, albeit theoretical in the absence of long-term data.

There is some evidence to support the use of tamoxifen prior to bicalutamide use or on development of breast symptoms. Surgical options include: adenomammectomy with periareolar incision; and incision and liposuction.

Bone health. Loss of bone mineral density (BMD) with ADT for prostate cancer is well recognized, with significant loss of BMD occurring within 12 months of starting therapy: the annual loss is approximately 2–8% per year at the lumbar spine and 2–6% at the hip. The loss appears to continue indefinitely while treatment continues, and there is no recovery after therapy ceases. Just under 20% of men surviving at least 5 years after a diagnosis of prostate cancer have a fracture if treated with ADT compared with around 13% of men not receiving this therapy; this is equivalent to one additional fracture for every 28 men treated with ADT.

Vitamin D deficiency exacerbates the development of osteoporosis, so vitamin D status should be evaluated before commencing ADT in men with prostate cancer.

Bisphosphonates (zoledronic acid [zoledronate], pamidronic acid [pamidronate] and alendronic acid [alendronate]) in men treated with ADT have been shown to prevent bone loss in prospective studies and to increase BMD in one randomized controlled trial; bisphosphonates have also been shown to reduce the incidence of skeletal-related events in men with prostate cancer. Further prospective trials are required to assess the efficacy and cost-effectiveness of bisphosphonates in men with prostate cancer who require ADT. Until the results from these trials become available, suggestions for the management of bone effects in men treated with ADT include baseline and yearly measurements of BMD. Baseline calcium, phosphate, liver function, thyroid function, 25-hydroxy vitamin D and parathyroid hormone assays should be performed, and calcium and vitamin D supplementation as well as isometric exercises, should be encouraged. Osteonecrosis of the mandible is a rare complication of bisphosphonate therapy.

Metabolic syndrome and cardiovascular risk. Metabolic syndrome is a constellation of cardiovascular risk factors (e.g. fasting hyperglycemia, hypertriglycerolemia, decreased serum HDL-cholesterol, increases in waist circumference, increased waist to hip ratio and hypertension) that have been reported to be elevated in men receiving ADT.

The first study to report an increase in cardiovascular risk for men treated with ADT was a retrospective study of 79 196 men in whom an increased risk of coronary disease, myocardial infarction and ventricular arrhythmia was identified. Another large retrospective study also suggested a 20% increase in cardiovascular morbidity with 1 year of ADT. A study by D'Amico et al. reported that in men older than 65, treatment with ADT decreases the time to fatal myocardial infarction compared with men not receiving this therapy. A large number of other studies have, however, failed to show any major differences in cardiovascular morbidity.

As this area is controversial, it is prudent to critically weigh the risks and benefits of ADT in men with cardiovascular risk factors. It is also important to monitor all the risk factors carefully in all men undergoing androgen deprivation and to treat these risk factors where appropriate.

Lipid profile. ADT alters lipid profiles, potentially increasing cardiovascular risk. Total cholesterol rises by approximately 10%, triacylglycerols by 25% and LDL-cholesterol by 7%. However, this may be counteracted by a reported 11% rise in HDL-cholesterol levels.

Insulin sensitivity is related to testosterone levels; ADT results in an 11–13% reduction in insulin sensitivity. A number of large studies have reported a 19–49% increase in the risk of developing diabetes mellitus in men receiving ADT.

Waist circumference increases while on ADT, but waist to hip ratio and hypertension have not been consistently reported in trials.

Management. Before ADT is started, a detailed medical examination and history should be taken, with particular focus on cardiac risk factors. This will enable proactive management before any condition becomes worsened as a consequence of ADT. Body weight, blood pressure, serum lipids and fasting blood glucose should be monitored regularly during ADT (at 3-monthly intervals from 3 months onward).

Key points – survivorship and treatment complications

- Men with prostate cancer require emotional support as well as information on probable outcomes and the effects of the disease and its treatment.
- Sexual dysfunction is a common sequela of prostate cancer treatment. An open and informed discussion with the patient and his partner will do much to counter anxiety and loss of self-esteem.
- Erectile dysfunction can often be improved with phosphodiesterase type 5 inhibitors, prostaglandin suppositories or injections, or mechanical vacuum devices.
- Loss of libido can be reduced by using antiandrogens as opposed to bilateral orchidectomy or a luteinizing hormone-releasing hormone (LHRH) analog to treat prostate cancer.
- Osteoporosis and fractures are side effects of long-term androgen deprivation therapy (ADT): vitamin D status should be evaluated before starting ADT, and calcium and vitamin D supplementation, as well as isometric exercises, encouraged during treatment.
- It is prudent to weigh the risks and benefits of ADT in men with cardiovascular risk factors and to monitor all risk factors during therapy. At-risk patients should be advised to make lifestyle changes as appropriate (e.g. stop smoking, lose weight).

Patients at risk should be advised to make lifestyle changes before and while using ADT:

- stop smoking
- lose weight if necessary
- eat a healthy diet.

Individual risk factors should be actively managed – for example, lipid-lowering agents for hyperlipidemia and glucose-lowering agents for diabetes.

Key references

Alibhai SM, Duong-Hua M, Sutradhar R et al. Impact of androgen deprivation therapy on cardiovascular disease and diabetes. *J Clin Oncol* 2009;27:3452–8.

Carson C, McMahon CG. *Fast Facts: Erectile Dysfunction*, 4th edn. Oxford: Health Press Ltd, 2008.

D'Amico AV, Denham JW, Crook J et al. Influence of androgen suppression therapy for prostate cancer on the frequency and timing of fatal myocardial infarctions. *J Clin Oncol* 2007;25:2420–5.

Holmes-Walker DJ, Woo H, Gurney H et al. Maintaining bone health in patients with prostate cancer. *Med J Aust* 2006;184:176–9.

Levine GN, D'Amico AV, Berger P et al. Androgen-deprivation therapy in prostate cancer and cardiovascular risk: a science advisory from the American Heart Association, American Cancer Society, and American Urological Association: endorsed by the American Society for Radiation Oncology. *Circulation* 2010;121:833–40.

Montorsi F, Guazzoni G, Strambi LF et al. Recovery of spontaneous erectile function after nerve-sparing radical retropubic prostatectomy with and without early intracavernous injections of alprostadil: results of a prospective, randomized trial. *J Urol* 1997;58:1408–10.

Montorsi F, Nathan HP, McCullough A et al. Tadalafil in the treatment of erectile dysfunction following bilateral nerve sparing radical retropubic prostatectomy: a randomized, double-blind, placebo controlled trial. *J Urol* 2004;172:1036–41.

Penson DF, McLerran D, Feng Z et al. 5-year urinary and sexual outcomes after radical prostatectomy: results from the Prostate Cancer Outcomes Study. *J Urol* 2008;179(suppl):S40–4.

Saad F, Adachi JD, Brown JP et al. Cancer treatment-induced bone loss in breast and prostate cancer. *J Clin Oncol* 2008;26:5465–76.

Saigal CS, Gore JL, Krupski TL et al. Androgen deprivation therapy increases cardiovascular morbidity in men with prostate cancer. *Cancer* 2007;110:1493–500.

Scher HI, Fizazi K, Saad F et al. Increased survival with enzalutamide in prostate cancer after chemotherapy. *N Engl J Med* 2012;367:1187–97.

Slack A, Newman DK, Wein AJ. *Fast Facts: Bladder Disorders*, 2nd edn. Oxford: Health Press Ltd, 2011.

Smith MR, Finkelstein JS, McGovern FJ et al. Changes in body composition during androgen deprivation therapy for prostate cancer. *J Clin Endocrinol Metab* 2002;87:599–603.

Smith MR, Lee H, McGovern F et al. Metabolic changes during gonadotropin-releasing hormone agonist therapy for prostate cancer: differences from the classic metabolic syndrome. *Cancer* 2008;112:2188–94.

Smith MR, Lee H, Nathan DM. Insulin sensitivity during combined androgen blockade for prostate cancer. *J Clin Endocrinol Metab* 2006;91:1305–8.

Useful resources

UK

Macmillan Cancer Support
Tel: +44 (0)20 7840 7840
Helpline: 0808 808 00 00
www.macmillan.org.uk

Men's Health Forum
Tel: +44 (0)20 7922 7908
www.menshealthforum.org.uk

Prostate Cancer Research Centre
Tel: +44 (0)20 7679 9366
www.prostate-cancer-research.org.uk

Prostate Cancer UK
Tel: +44 (0)20 3310 7000
Helpline: 0800 074 8383
prostatecanceruk.org

USA

American Cancer Society
Toll-free: 1 800 227 2345
www.cancer.org

American Urological Association
Toll-free: 1 866 746 4282
www.auanet.org

National Cancer Institute
Toll-free: 1 800 422 6237
www.cancer.gov/cancertopics/types/prostate

Prostate Cancer Foundation
Tel: +1 310 570 4700
Toll-free: 1 800 757 2873
www.pcf.org

Prostate Cancer Research Institute
Tel: +1 310 743 2116
Helpline: 1 800 641 7274
www.prostate-cancer.org

Prostate Conditions Education Council
Tel: +1 303 316 4685
Toll-free: 1 866 477 6788
www.prostateconditions.org

ZERO – The End of Prostate Cancer
Tel: +1 202 463 9455
Toll-free: 1 888 245 9455
www.zerocancer.org

International

Prostate Cancer Canada
Tel: +1 416 441 2131
Toll-free: 1 888 255 0333
www.prostatecancer.ca

Prostate Cancer Foundation of Australia
Tel: +61 (0)2 9438 7000
Toll-free: 1800 220 099
www.prostate.org.au

Other useful websites

Cancer Research UK
www.cancerresearchuk.org

Embarrassing Problems
www.embarrassingproblems.com

Hormone-Refractory Prostate Cancer
www.hrpca.org

James Buchanan Brady Urological Institute
urology.jhu.edu

Johns Hopkins Medicine
www.hopkinsmedicine.org

Marie Curie Cancer Care
www.mariecurie.org.uk

Mayo Clinic prostate cancer
www.mayoclinic.com/health/prostate-cancer/DS00043

Memorial Sloan-Kettering Cancer Center
www.mskcc.org

Patient Pictures
www.patientpictures.com/urology

William Catalona
(developer of the PSA test)
www.drcatalona.com

Further reading – fastfacts.com

Other *Fast Facts* titles that may be of interest include:
Fast Facts: Benign Prostatic Hyperplasia
Fast Facts: Bladder Disorders
Fast Facts: Depression
Fast Facts: Erectile Dysfunction
Fast Facts: Obesity

Index

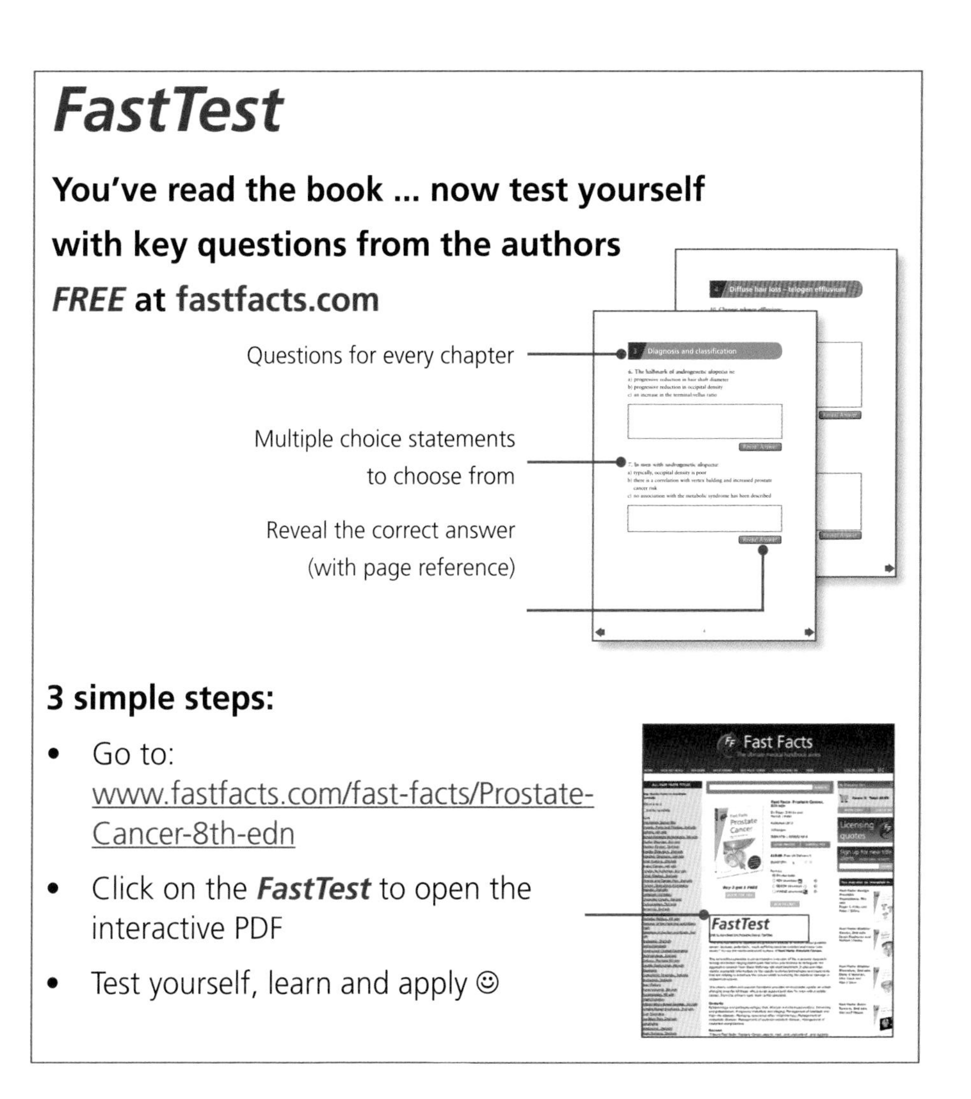
FastTest
You've read the book ... now test yourself
with key questions from the authors
FREE at fastfacts.com
Questions for every chapter
Multiple choice statements
to choose from
Reveal the correct answer
(with page reference)
3 simple steps:
Go to:
www.fastfacts.com/fast-facts/Prostate-Cancer-8th-edn
Click on the FastTest to open the interactive PDF
Test yourself, learn and apply ☺
Fast Facts
FastTest

FF Fast Facts

The ultimate medical handbook series

Our hope is that this Fast Facts *title helps you to improve your practice and, in turn, improves the health of your patients*

What will you do next?

Use this space to write some action points that have come from reading this book and testing yourself. And don't worry if you pass this on to a colleague, senior or junior; they are bound to find them interesting and may wish to add their own.

Action Point 1

Action Point 2

Action Point 3

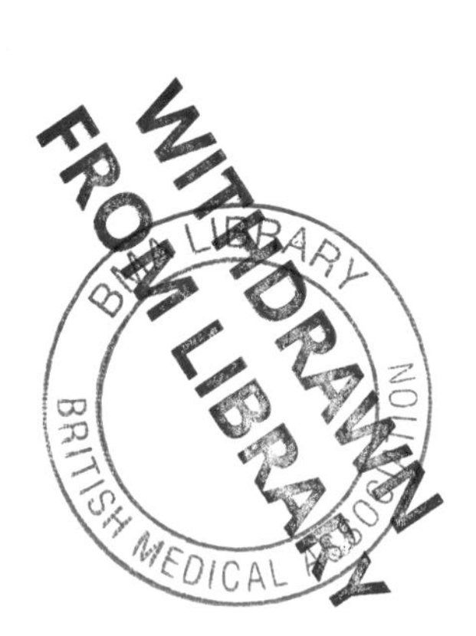

If you have the time to share them with us, or you have suggestions of how to improve the next edition, we'd love to hear from you at **feedback@fastfacts.com**